The nurses' handbook

By Ann Jaloba with interviews
by Jean Gray

The nurses' handbook

The nurses' handbook

ISBN-13: 978-0-9954599-0-8

Published by Ann Jaloba Publishing, 26 Tapton Mount Close, Sheffield S10 5DJ

The nurses' handbook

THIS BOOK IS DEDICATED TO

All the nurses we have met over the years who have made this book possible. Thank you

Ann Jaloba and Jean Gray

The nurses' handbook

A quick hello from the people you will meet in this book

We thought you might want to find out a bit more

about us and all our contributors. So here goes . . .

Ann Jaloba

is a writer and publisher and also a practising therapist, using hypnotherapy and neuro linguistic programming to help her clients reach their full potential

Jean Gray

worked for many years for the publishing company of the Royal College of Nursing. She has recently been involved in the Mary Seacole Memorial Statue Appeal

Christine Hancock

was the General Secretary of the Royal College of Nursing, 1989–2001. She is the founder and director of the global health charity C3 Collaborating for Health

Elizabeth Anionwu CBE

is Emeritus Professor of Nursing, University of West London and Vice Chair, Mary Seacole Memorial Statue Appeal. She has recently written her autobiography *Mixed Blessings from a Cambridge Union*.

Fiona Murphy

is Assistant Director of Nursing, Bereavement & Donor Support, Salford, Bolton & Wigan NHS Foundation Trusts

Laura Downes

spent may years in nursing journalism, latterly as Group Educational Projects Manager, RCNi, formerly RCN Publishing

Jean White

is Chief Nursing Officer for Wales/Nurse Director NHS Wales, and a visiting professor to the University of South Wales and Cardiff University

Paul Jebb

is Experience of Care Professional lead, NHS England

Tara Beaumont

recently retired from her role as a MacMillan nurse and now manages a gardening business with her husband

CONTENTS

Get extra resources. Set up a readers' club.

More details and your special password on

page 201

the nurses' handbook

Foreword

By Christine Hancock

Nursing is a fantastic job. For many people work is not especially interesting or rewarding, but it pays wages and provides company; but nurses rarely go home saying they had a boring day or wonder if there is any value in the work they do. Every day, nurses walk into people's lives and know they make a difference.

Nursing is also a hard and challenging job: faced every day with pain, suffering, bereavement in a way that few others experience.

It can be especially frustrating and distressing to know that with more time, more staff, more resources, you could have made someone more comfortable, less anxious, or helped a frightened or grieving relative to face a difficult reality. Then, at the end of a shift, many nurses cannot go home and find themselves cared for and pampered, but often looking after needy children, partners or elderly family members.

So it is good to find a book focused not on nursing but on nurses themselves. Nurses, of course, work in a variety of settings, although often it seems that the media only focuses attention on busy acute hospitals. There are different challenges in the different aspects of various workplaces; the pressure of fast turnover in acute hospital settings, the complaints of people kept waiting in emergency departments, the loneliness of people cared for at home, working with the grumpiness of a tired doctor, the fear of error in operating rooms, the tight staffing and low wages of care homes. All have their pressures, their challenges and their rewards. This book offers something for all nurses wherever they work.

The book concentrates on you, a nurse, and what you need just for yourself: your own health: a healthy diet, managing shift systems and their effect on your sleep; the different pressures be they stress, bullying or the nature of the clinical care. It offers practical help and guidance so you can help yourself, or know where to turn to, and what your rights are in various situations.

A career in nursing may last for forty years, but it is unlikely to be the same job throughout that time: technology and science will change the job, your own family circumstances, age and health will change you and what you want from work. In addressing career guidance, the book provides a helpful and practical way of offering nurses the chance to think about ways to continue to use their qualifications and skills while exploring new options or just having a break from one environment.

A book such as this can be important as a way to offer nurses ideas about how to manage the challenge of their working life, where help and advice might be found, and what alternatives are available. My concern is whether busy nurses will find this book? Will they have time to read it? Will they be able to act upon the ideas, advice and suggestions that could be important to them? Perhaps groups of nurses might share it? Each concentrating on one or two aspects and use it to stimulate discussion. However used, this book offers each nurse the opportunity to reflect on her/himself on their work, on the current job and on the future. Every nurse can feel confident in her/his future.

Christine Hancock

the nurses' handbook

Introduction
by Ann Jaloba and Jean Gray

Ann says:

Do you ever notice that however carefully you plan your next move something else can come along and change your direction? The genesis of this book has been an example of this, and in a very good way. It has felt as if various interests and experiences I have had over my working life have come together and the result has been this book.

So let me explain a bit about myself. I work as a hypnotherapist, using a mixture of hypnotherapy, neuro-linguistic programming and coaching techniques to help people reach their full potential and optimum wellbeing. This feels like a great way to make a living; I get to spend every day being given insight into other people's lives and helping them change. It is completely fulfilling and makes me very happy.

I've been doing this for seven years now. I work mainly in Sheffield, just up the road from four NHS hospitals and very near numerous private hospitals, clinics and nursing homes. That's where things began to change for me. I never planned to specialise in helping nurses when I started on this path, but, given where I practise, it is not surprising that so many of my clients are nurses. I have a pretty good success record with the nurses who come to see me, probably because I know a fair bit about their experiences as I am not new to the world of health care. I was deputy editor of *Nursing Standard* back in the 1990s and website manager at the Royal College of Nursing in the early part of this century. I have been able to call on the knowledge and networks I had built up in the nursing world to help the nurse clients who now come though my door.

As I built up something of a reputation for helping nurses and other health professionals deal with the ups and downs of work and life, I began to focus even more on how the techniques and skills I had gained as a hypnotherapist and as a hypnotherapy supervisor could help nurses achieve optimum career and life satisfaction and well being.

Over the years I have acquired a toolkit of helpful techniques, knowledge, stories and research which I give my nurse clients to help with conditions such as stress and burnout. I have also coached nurses who want to take a different career step and helped with specific problems such as bullying at work, making career changes and deciding which field of nursing best suits a particular client.

One person I had always kept up with from my days at *Nursing Standard* was the former editor, my great friend and colleague Jean Gray. She had trained as a counsellor, so we frequently spoke about talking therapies and how they could help health professionals. Over time we developed the idea of using all this knowledge, anecdote and experience for this book and here it is.

As a nurse you will often have been told to look after yourself so you can look after others. I hope this book makes that phrase very real for you and encourages you to put yourself first for once as well.

My aim in the book is to help you help yourself by giving you enough background and enough techniques and ideas so you will have options next time you hit a rough patch, or want to make a change and develop in a new direction.

I start with a firmly-held belief in what are known as 'solution-focused therapies'. The key thing about this group of therapies is the understanding that you have the resources to make good choices. Through guided questioning and intervention and working to refine your mindset, you can come up with what is right for you.

You do not have to do this in isolation. Luckily, we are living through a time where there has been a big, and to my way of thinking very welcome, change in how we think about our mental health and general wellbeing.

For some time now (going back to the middle of the last century) there has been a strand in psychology which, rather than looking at what happens when things go wrong with people's mental health, looks at what happens when things are going well. This has developed and deepened and formed the basis of solution-focused approaches and therapies.

So we start from the point of view that as long as we are alive we are doing things, making decisions, taking actions. We cannot *not* do this, even if we are lying in bed with the duvet over our heads that is still a choice, an action, a doing (and sometimes it may even be a good choice).

So, if you are always making choices and doing things which create your life experience, why not make sure you are making the best possible choices and doing the best possible things for you? And if you think about it there is so much that you do well - I bet you do much more well than you do badly. A good place to start is with those areas where you feel accomplished, happy and at peace with yourself. Look at and celebrate those areas and then ask yourself how you do this, pay close attention to how you make your own success. Then you can see if you can replicate these behaviours and habits of thought in areas which feel more difficult and challenging for you. You can also look at it from the other side. If you are miserable, then what are you doing to create or exacerbate this? This is not to say that everything is your fault, it is not. Bad things do happen to good people. But it is to say that when those bad things happen there are often ways to control and change how you feel about them and how you react to them and this can be learned.

This is not to buy into the myth that we can all do anything. That just isn't true and often the world around us creates pressures and stresses which we have to deal with. And there are few places where this is truer than in the health services. Changing demographics, changing attitudes in society, the increasing chance that your performance is constantly measured and cuts in resources, can all make your job, and therefore your life, feel harder. On top of this, we all live with a rapid pace of change, and change and uncertainty can be uncomfortable.

Keeping well in the real world
The book is designed with you and your working environment in mind. I suggest things you can do which acknowledge that you will often be very stretched and overworked, that you have other responsibilities outside of work and that you work in what can be very difficult circumstances. The very things which make nursing such a

18

fulfilling career are also what make it such a demanding one. Dealing with people when they are frightened, in pain and face life-changing or life-limiting circumstances is tough and can take an emotional toll. I hope in this book I give you some ways to protect yourself so you can give the best to your patients and to yourself.

I would like to think that after you have read this book you will have many ways to look after yourself, not just today but in the years which lie ahead. So I have given you a lot of techniques and exercises to help your wellbeing (and you can find more on the book's website www.nursesbook.com) but I have also tried to explain the theories behind these ideas and how they came about. Hopefully you will gain the confidence to adapt these techniques in ways that suit you. There is no magic, many of them are common sense and all can be improved with your input to make them work for you. The book will help you protect yourself from the unavoidable pressures and structures of a nursing life, so I cover things such as coping with burnout, dealing with shift patterns and getting the most out of clinical supervision.

The book is not there just to help you deal with problems, but also to develop your full potential. My aim is to help you make the most of the huge diversity of career possibilities within nursing and I suggest how you can make good career choices based on the type of person you are. I hope I can help you build an optimistic, healthy outward-looking mindset which will stand you in good stead through both the good and bad times. Finally, we now understand more about how closely mental and physical wellbeing are linked, so I make some suggestions about how you can eat as healthily as possible, even when the food around you is not the best, and you will find some tips that can help you build exercise and physical activity

into your life however busy you are.
I hope you enjoy this book and find it helpful. I am delighted constantly at how wonderful nearly all the nurses I meet think nursing is. The nurses Jean has interviewed telling such varied stories are yet another reflection of this and I loved reading their stories.

Jean adds:

Although I had met and worked with nearly all of the nurses interviewed in this book - some over many years, others on specific projects – the experience of talking to them about the sweep of their professional lives was an eye-opener and a truly enjoyable one.

I would like to thank all of them for their enthusiasm, their willingness to talk openly about their experiences and most of all for their generosity in taking time to talk to me. I believe they did so because they know that nursing can be tough, but it is also wonderfully rewarding and they never tire of sharing that passion with others.

All are successful in their fields of practice and while they may be at different stages in their careers, I was struck by one major theme that came through in their stories: they may be high achievers, but all had suffered set backs at various points along the way. However, they share the wisdom to know when a work situation is no longer right for them, and they all found the courage to move on. So if you take one message from reading about these nursing role models, I hope it will be that the techniques developed by Ann Jaloba can help you to achieve the same wisdom and courage.

Each of these role models has their own story to tell about how they came into nursing; their career paths have been many and varied. But the good news is that all have great faith in modern nursing and have no hesitation in recommending the profession to future generations - with one caveat. As Jean White puts it: "More than anything, you need to care about other people, to understand that it is a privilege to do this work. That will come across in how you think and how you deal with people." Nursing offers a huge variety of opportunities across many settings that can satisfy all sorts of personalities - introvert and extrovert, those who need instant rewards for their efforts compared with others who are in for the long haul. However, no matter which path your nursing career takes, the core values of caring and compassion underpin everything. And that includes taking care of yourself. I hope this book will help you get the best from the wonderful career choice you made.

the nurses' handbook

Chapter One
The big picture: you can teach yourself to be happy

If you want to arrive at your destination then it helps to

know where you want to go and have a good map to

get you there. So let us start with the big questions.

What makes us happy and how can we achieve that?

I am going to share a lot of ideas throughout this book. I hope these will help you deal with the everyday challenges, problems and ups and downs of your life as a nurse. Before we get down to that level of detail though, let's soar above the fray and look at the big picture.

Thought experiment: bird's eye view
Try this thought experiment. Imagine you can fly, perhaps see yourself as a majestic bird soaring and swooping on the air currents.

Now image you are flying above a landscape – you can see it below and as you watch you realise you are looking down on scenes from your life: past, present and possibly future. As you watch your life from this high vantage point, notice what is in the clearest focus.

What seems to stand out for you? It could be friends, or family, or your work. All these things and more will probably be there but what is the clearest for you?

Doing this exercise often makes people feel good. Floating above everything and the perspective it gives you can create a sensation of great freedom and understanding. Enjoy what you are experiencing; there is no right or wrong here, just a way to gain some insight into your values.

When you feel you have done as much as feels comfortable for you, or as much as you have time for, let yourself come back gently to earth again and reflect on what has happened.

Do you feel you can now answer the question: 'what do I want to achieve in my life?' The answer you give will be unique to you. If it seems too difficult to answer at the moment, then try pondering on these common values.

- Do you want to be happy?
- Do you want to have a fulfilled life?
- Do you want to be useful?

Your wishes could include any or all of these. If it is all these things, ask yourself which feels *to you* to be the most important?

Or you might have found that what you want is something very different from the list above, and that is fine too. You know yourself best and what you come up with will be the most valid for you. At this early stage, you may not be entirely sure of what a fulfilled and happy life would look like for you, but you will have a pretty good idea about the sort of things which matter most to you. You will know instinctively what those are.

I am going to start with a presumption that whatever you come up with is right for you. So trust yourself.

These instincts are your starting point and they are rarely wrong, but often they can get lost or submerged in the rough and tumble of day-to-day life. Now let's underpin those instincts with some facts, some evidence and some theory.

What makes us happy: the new science
I am going to begin by looking at how some thinkers have answered the question of what makes a happy and fulfilled life. Luckily, we are dealing with these questions at a time when our understanding of how we live our emotional and spiritual lives has come on leaps and bounds with the development of the set of ideas known as positive psychology, or the science of happiness.

These ideas grew up in the latter half of the 20th century and are still being refined and developed into the 21st. They focus on what makes a happy, meaningful, successful or fulfilled life rather than looking at the roots of mental illness. One of the best-known protagonists of these ideas, Martin Seligman, describes it in his book *Authentic Happiness*. Positive psychology, he says: "takes you through the countryside of pleasure and gratification, up into the high country of strength and virtue, and finally to the peaks of lasting fulfilment, meaning and purpose."

Prior to this, psychology and investigations into mental health and well-being tended generally to work from a model that assumed people had something wrong with them which needed fixing and once the fix was applied everything would be fine. These models began with a problem and focused on how it could be overcome.

The thinkers we will be looking at moved away from this to concentrate on what happens when people lead happy and fulfilling lives and what we can learn from this to optimise human potential.

As the Austrian psychologist Marie Jahoda put it in her 1958 book *Current Concepts of Positive Mental Health*: "the absence of mental illness is not a sufficient indicator of mental health." This way of looking at the world does not deny that some of us, perhaps all of us, will have problems in our lives, but it *does* look at why some of us seem to cope better than others. It concentrates on what happens, what we are doing, when things go well. (And remember, we can never do nothing, whether we are creating a happy or a sad life we are the actors in our own constantly unfolding drama.) This set of theories and techniques say that happiness or living a meaningful life is a mindset or a habit. It asks the questions: "how do happy people 'do' their happiness – and what is happiness anyway?". For example, Martin Seligman believes it is possible to learn happiness and this can be a massive benefit to people who are depressed or unhappy.

How do we 'do' happiness?
So how do we 'do' happiness? If we can understand this, and there is now serious and extensive scientific research into the area, then it should be possible to teach it, to replicate it, so we can learn to repeat what we do when things go well. We should also have a way of helping people who are down, depressed or unhappy in some way by coaching them in how they can behave differently.

I am going to quickly run through how this way of thinking developed, what its main theorists had to say and how they applied their theories in practical terms.

Viktor Frankl: finding meaning in the worst of circumstances
Let's begin with the work of Viktor Frankl, an Austrian neurologist who had lived through terrible experiences in the 2nd World War.

Frankl was Jewish and spent much of the war in Nazi work camps. In this time, he developed a firm philosophy that each person is fundamentally healthy and has the resources they need to live a fulfilled life. His best known book *Man's Search for Meaning* chronicles his experience of giving healthcare to his fellow prisoners. He observed that those who kept a sense of purpose and meaning in life survived longer than those who lost their belief that life had any purpose at all.

Viktor and his sister were the only members of the family who survived. After the war he returned to Vienna where he wrote *Man's Search for Meaning* although its German title, translated as *Saying Yes to Life in Spite of Everything, A Psychologist Experiences the Concentration Camp* probably sums it up better.

If meaning gives fulfilment to life, Frankl also believed that lack of meaning was a strong component in mental disorders, addictive behaviours and depression. As he put it: "Those who have a 'why' to live can bear with almost any 'how'." He believed that, even when faced with the most horrendous of circumstances, it was still within human capacity, the last human freedom, to choose one's attitude to one's circumstances.

He understood the importance of the work/life balance way before the term became fashionable, noting that some people experienced feelings of discontent, apathy and lack of motivation when their everyday work was finished. Work was important, indeed Frankl noted that animals who had tasks lived longer than those that did not, but the truly meaningful life needs more than work.

For Frankl, the meaningful life could be broken into three essential areas which took into account the uniqueness of every human being:
- *Doing*, using our talents in work or in other ways
- *Experiencing* the world through relationships, enjoyment of art and culture and the environment
- *Attitude*, which we always have the freedom to change whatever our circumstances. However, he did not believe there was a general answer to the question of life's meaning.

Frankl was a great believer in the individual making

choices for themselves. He said each individual's response to what life throws up would lead to each person finding their life's meaning for themselves through the choices they make. Frankl called his body of ideas logotherapy (from the Greek word logos meaning "meaning"). Some techniques based on Frankl's work are still in wide use today. Here are two very popular ones:

Dereflection

We are all familiar with the experience of being unable to stop thinking about a problem or issue, we keep turning it over in our minds and everything else seems to fade into the background. Meanwhile, the problem continues to go around and around in our heads.

In this state we frequently become self-obsessed, constantly concerned with how we look and behave and what others think of us. Of course this can make our problem worse; it can even become difficult to carry out everyday tasks. Frankl developed the dereflection technique to help us in such situations.

He advised taking the focus away from oneself and making the effort to reflect instead on the task at hand. By losing oneself in a task or an experience our attention is diverted from ourselves, we lose the focus on ourselves and by doing so actually find ourselves again. You can use this technique for yourself, and you will see many examples in this book. Here is one you can do anytime.

Help yourself: focus on a task

If you are having a bad day at work then find a task you know you must do and which will take you between a few minutes and half an hour.

Start that task as soon as you can, and really focus on

what you are doing, keeping the task in the forefront of your mind.
You can do this even if it is a routine task which you normally would not need to think about.

Talk to yourself, (silently if there are others around) describing what you are doing at every step. Imagine you are explaining it to an alien from another planet. With this sort of focus you will notice new things about the task.

When your attention drifts, gently bring it back to the task.
However often your attention drifts, bring it back. At the end you will feel as if you have had a little holiday from your worries. You may even have found a new way to do that routine task - but that's a bonus.

***

Paradoxical intention
Frankl noticed that we can spend lots of time worrying about things which actually never happen. So he developed a way of dealing with this, which can be summed up as: "It's never as bad as what you fear." He suggested that you ask: how would it be if you deliberately wished for what you feared might happen? What if you created that feared thing deliberately? Do this and the anticipatory anxiety of worrying about the thing you fear would go.

If you have ever found yourself feeling anxious about your anxiety, obsessing about the symptoms of that anxiety and then psychologically or even physically fleeing from what is making you anxious, then you will have noticed those thoughts and actions are anxiety-inducing in themselves.

The more we try to fight the fear, the stronger the fear

becomes. This technique short-circuits that process. Here is an example of how I used it with a nurse client of mine.

Case study: Helen's nightmare handover

One of my clients, Helen, had this problem and this is what we did. There was one particular colleague who upset Helen because she felt he never listened to her and sniggered when she hesitated as she delivered the ward handover.

I asked her to imagine doing the handover, but rather than just hesitating she was to imagine stuttering and losing her place and having to go back to the beginning. The unpleasant colleague was laughing out loud and others were joining in.
She concentrated on reading the handover as badly as she possibly could. She worked at making her mouth dry, her breathing fast and her sweating worse. She paid attention to how she did this. I kept prompting her to tell me what she was doing. At the end she understood that she created this situation by taking some definite actions.

She knew now what she did, and it was her doing it, to create the failed handover. Because she had created the anxiety she could uncreate it. She could stop it. And she could approach the activity differently. She might still hesitate, but that was okay. I convinced Helen of this by adding a third technique, derived from Frankl, known as Socratic questioning. By asking simple questions about her expectations and beliefs she could be gently guided to understand that the way she conceived of the handover was unhelpful and not reflective of the actual situation. This took

*the level of fear down a notch and made it easier for her to
cope.*

***

**Abraham Maslow and Erich Fromm: happiness in the real
world**
Another thinker who is important to our story is Abraham
Maslow. The term positive psychology was first coined by him
and he achieved fantastic insight into what had to happen for
us to feel fulfilled by our work.

Maslow was born in New York and has spent his career
investigating what he calls self-actualisation. He studied two
colleagues whom he admired, an anthropologist called Ruth
Benedict and a Gestalt psychologist called Max Wertheimer,
to see if he could discover what it was that made them
successful and fulfilled individuals. He was also influenced by
the work of Erich Fromm, who was active and influential in
the second half of the 20th century.

Fromm was also concerned with how humans coped in
modern society. He believed that modern, increasingly
bureaucratic and stratified societies were stopping people
realising their essential social and connected nature. Fromm
believed modern society was in danger of blocking the
essential social nature of the human being. In his book, *The
Art of Loving* (1956) he said:

"Our society is run by a managerial bureaucracy, by
professional politicians; people are motivated by mass
suggestion, their aim is producing more and consuming more,
as purposes in themselves. All activities are subordinated to
economic goals, means have become ends; man is an
automaton — well fed, well clad, but without any ultimate
concern for that which is his peculiarly human quality and
function. If man is to be able to love, he must be put in his

supreme place. The economic machine must serve him, rather than he serve it. He must be enabled to share experience, to share work, rather than, at best, share in profits. Society must be organized in such a way that man's social, loving nature is not separated from his social existence, but becomes one with it. If it is true, as I have tried to show, that love is the only sane and satisfactory answer to the problem of human existence, then any society which excludes, relatively, the development of love, must in the long run perish of its own contradiction with the basic necessities of human nature."

It was this focus on what it means to be human at its best and what it means to be human in society, especially through work, which interested Abraham Maslow. As he said, in his 1968 book *Towards a Psychology of Being*: "It is as if Freud supplied us the sick half of psychology and we must now fill it out with the healthy half."

One great thing about Maslow is that his writing reflects the lives most of us live in the real world, where we have to work to earn enough money to pay the mortgage or the rent and put food on the table.

And of course work is not always what we would want it to be. But in acknowledging that basic needs (for food, shelter etc.) must be fulfilled, Maslow also stressed that for humans to be fully human they needed more. In 1954, in his book *Motivation and Personality* he said:

"Human life will never be understood unless its highest aspirations are taken into account. Growth, self-actualization, the striving toward health, the quest for identity and autonomy, the yearning for excellence (and other ways of phrasing the striving 'upward') must by now be accepted beyond question as a widespread and perhaps universal human tendency. . ."

As with the other thinkers we have been looking at,

32

Maslow was interested in what was going on when things went well for people, rather than focusing on problems. He believed that people are motivated by what they want to achieve. Maslow's best-known idea is the hierarchy of needs, which has been used a lot in management theory. The hierarchy is usually represented in the form of a pyramid. At the bottom sit basic physical needs, things we must do to keep alive, such as eating, drinking and breathing. These must be fulfilled first, before people do anything else and if they are not fulfilled nothing else matters – people become completely preoccupied with satisfying them.

Next comes the need for basic safety and security. This includes protection from the elements, and from predators. It also includes those things which are needed for security in the modern world, such as ability to pay the rent or mortgage and to have a reasonably secure job.

The next layer is the need to belong: to a family; a group of friends or a community. Both the safety and security and the belonging layer reflect the need to build resilience. If these needs are fulfilled then we can be resilient to the knocks and changes which come in every life.

The next two layers are about how we as individuals can develop to our maximum potential.

So the fourth layer focuses on esteem which Maslow argues comes from doing what one does in life well: being competent, taking responsibility and getting recognition for doing so. However, Maslow was clear that true self-esteem does not come simply from the approval of others, indeed only seeking the approval of others can lead to psychological problems as there can be a dissonance between your feelings and the world around you. People with low self-esteem often crave respect from others; they may even feel the need to seek fame or glory. However, fame or glory will not help build self-esteem. Maslow describes self-esteem as an inner core of confidence in which we truly can enjoy our successes and achievements.

The layer at the very top of the hierarchy is self-actualisation. Maslow has pondered long on and written much about this concept.

At its heart lies creativity and achieving the very best for and of oneself. Maslow studied people he felt had reached this point and noted that, whether rich or poor, whether others would have regarded them as successful or not, they shared some common characteristics. This is what he found about these people:

- They are honest with themselves, seeing things as they are
- They accept themselves and others, including flaws, humouring and tolerating faults and they can laugh at themselves
- They are self-reliant and make their own judgements
- They look outside of themselves and become engrossed in tasks and projects which they regard as valuable

You may think that these characteristics are those which make a good nurse. It may be that some of the role models you have or some of the colleagues you admire have these traits. If so, take a closer look at what they do and ask if you could model their behaviour. This does not mean copying everything they do, but rather looking at the attitude with which they do it.

Maslow's concepts can be a great guide here. You may notice something else as well: those people who seem very happy in their work, and in the rest of their lives, often seem to do things effortlessly. Maslow believed this characteristic of self- actualisers and that they experience something he called 'peak experiences'.

In *Towards a Psychology of Being* he described peak experience as functioning effortlessly and without any fear or inhibition, being mindful and in the present and whole and harmonious. You will probably be able to think of at least a few occasions when you have felt this. Take a little time and see if you can work out common factors at work during those times. Then ask if you can do this more often. That would be good wouldn't it?

Csikszentmihalyi and 'flow'

This focus on what it means to be at our best was also investigated by the Hungarian writer Mihaly Csikszentmihalyi. He used his own experience to identify a state of mind which he called 'flow'. This was a state where the person became engaged in activity to the extent that it absorbed them completely. He noticed that this was a state experienced by people engaged in creative activities, but importantly, he noted that it came from *attitude* rather than the external nature of a task.

I have often used this insight to help clients who are feeling very stressed or are depressed, so it's worth telling you a little more about this concept. Csikszentmihalyi noted two people doing a similar job could experience it differently. One could consider it fun while another found it a chore.

As he said in his 1992 work *Flow: the Psychology of Optimal Experience*: "So we have to assume that it is not what people do that counts but how they do it. Being an engineer or a carpenter is not in itself enjoyable. But if one does these things in a certain way then they become intrinsically rewarding, worth doing for their own sake."

Later, he conducted research into the state of mind of teenagers and found that when they were deeply involved in challenging tasks they reported a more upbeat mood. Csikszentmihalyi studied people who did things for enjoyment but with no immediate prospect of external reward and asked what was going on. He found: "It was clear

from talking to them that what kept them motivated was the quality of experience they felt when they were involved with the activity. This feeling didn't come when they were relaxing, when they were taking drugs or alcohol, or when they were consuming the expensive privileges of wealth. Rather, it often involved painful, risky, difficult activities that stretched the person's capacity and involved an element of novelty and discovery. This optimal experience is what I have called flow because many of the respondents described the feeling when things were going well as an almost automatic, effortless, yet highly focused state of consciousness."
He identified these key elements:

- clear goals
- immediate feedback (we know how well we are doing)
- a merging of actions and awareness (we are totally focused on what we are doing)
- no distractions
- no worry about failure
- no self consciousness
- a distorted sense of time (it can seem that things take more or less time, the outside clock seems to disappear)
- the activity is an end in itself, enjoyable in itself.

Help yourself: memory lane

Try this if you want to remind yourself of what it is like to be in that flow. A good start is to remember when you were in this state. Everyone has experienced this at some time, often in childhood.

Think back to a sunny day in the school holidays, or remember running out of school at the end of the day. Or perhaps you played a game or loved swimming, or you

might remember sitting quietly drawing or reading. Just let
your mind drift back to that time and remember, get that
feeling of excitement coursing through your body.

That feels good in itself doesn't it?

Now think about what you can do in your adult life to
recreate this. It can be anything from adult colouring books
(very popular at the moment) to a brisk walk, or you might
take up a sport or begin a challenge. It is amazing how
quickly making just this one change can lift your mood.

***

Martin Seligman: training yourself to cope and 'Grit'
The last thinker I want to consider in this chapter is Martin
Seligman, probably the best known contemporary thinker in
this field and the founder of the Positive Psychology Centre
at the University of Pennsylvania.

Seligman focuses, especially in his later work, on the
ability of human beings to deal with unpleasant feelings and
negative emotions by cultivating good thinking habits.

He argues that even people who may be naturally
disposed to anxiety can learn to cope. There will always be
some bad days, he says, but it is still possible to function well.
This outlook is sometimes summed up in the phrase: "you
are not in control of what happens but you are in control of
how you feel about it."

Seligman backs up his assertions with statistics, evidence
and experiments and offers practical advice.

One such is his ABC. As he puts it: "It is beliefs (B) about
an adversity (A) — and not the adversity itself — that cause
the consequent (C) feelings" This is a point of major insight
for most people: Emotions don't follow inexorably from

external events, but from what you think about those events. And you can actually change what you think."

So how do you change what you think? Seligman argues that this is largely a matter of habit and application.

Thinking is a habit like any other and with application you can train yourself into good habits. You can learn optimism. Seligman contrasts optimism with "learned helplessness", the notion that you cannot change anything.

One difference he notes in the two types of thinking is that those who have a helpless pessimistic outlook believe that a bad event is going to last forever and affect everything in the future. People with an optimistic nature are more likely to believe that a bad event is just one event, that they can do something about it and its negative consequences will pass.

He describes this as 'Grit', a mixture of passion, self-discipline and persistence. He also believes that altruism and acts of kindness can help the person doing the act. Carrying out acts of kindness directs our interest outside of ourselves and gives meaning to life.

Seligman's work has developed over the years, as he has refined his ideas and gone beyond the notion of happiness to investigate what makes people flourish (*Flourish* is a title of one of his recent books.) He says there are five factors which make up wellbeing which can be described by the acronym PERMA. They are:

• Positive emotion (this is subjective, only you know if the emotion you feel is positive)

• Engagement (again this is subjective and is when you are so absorbed you are focused on the subject which absorbs you, rather than on yourself)

• Relationships (those around you and their relation to you)

• Meaning (being part of something more than oneself)

• Achievement (this is important for its own sake, not for

any external benefits it brings)

Using all this as a nurse
That brings us to the end of this brief round up. You will probably already have noticed that many of the best characteristics of nursing as a profession are the meaningful, fulfilling, relationship-building things which the thinkers we have been looking at have identified as part of a good life.

You are in a profession which will almost certainly give you something which all of the thinkers we have been looking at have identified as components of happiness and fulfilment.

You have a role in the world which is meaningful and useful. On the other hand, it can be emotionally draining as you are faced with high and often painful emotions and behaviours from your patients or clients and their families and friends.

You will benefit immensely if you learn to protect and nurture yourself and build resilience and I am going to show you some ways you can do this, whatever the circumstances, in the rest of this book.

the nurses' handbook

Stories from a nursing life: Elizabeth Anionwu

"Sometimes step back and realise what is important"

Elizabeth Anionwu CBE never wanted to do anything

except nurse. Her focus and love for the profession

shines through. She identifies curiosity, courage, and

an ability to stand up for yourself as the qualities

which have kept her going in a long and illustrious

career.

When did you decide to become a nurse?
I was probably around the age of four or five. I was living in a convent and had very bad eczema. It got so bad that I would often go down to the sickbay, sometimes even be admitted. There was one woman there who I called the woman in white. In fact she was a nun who I later discovered was also a nurse, which is why she wore a white habit rather than black.

She used to do regular dressings on my very raw patches of eczema and what I liked about her was that she used distraction therapy. When it came to changing the dressing it could be quite painful. She knew how to distract me and make me laugh, often by using a rude word or something like that. She would just make me burst out laughing and then she whipped off the dressing. I just thought she was fantastic because I knew how painful it could be. She was such a lovely, warm person.

What was the appeal?
I wanted to be like the nun because she did something that could be very distressing and painful, but she handled it in such a way that it wasn't. It meant there was no fear and trepidation when I had to have my dressings changed.

How did you take the decision - alone, with help from friends, family or a careers adviser?
The decision was entirely my own, so much so that I had to resist people who wanted me to study medicine.

My school was a technical high school with three streams: the secretarial stream, nursing stream and university stream. At first, they wanted to put me totally into the university stream, but I was very determined that I wanted to be a nurse, obstinate you might say, so they agreed a compromise. I combined a bit of preparation for nursing while taking the course that prepared you for university.

Was it your first career or did you do something else first?
I left school at 16 and became a school nursing assistant, working in an infant welfare clinic in Wolverhampton. Two months into that my asthma got very bad, partly because of the `pea-souper` fogs. The medical officer for health rescued me and found me a post in a residential school for delicate children on the borders of Wolverhampton and Shropshire. I stayed there until I was 18 and ready to move to London to train as a nurse.

Did you consider any other careers? If so, what were they and why did you reject them?
No, I was very focused, only ever wanted to be a nurse.

Did you have an image or fantasy about what nursing would be like?

Certainly, initially, it was based on the nun, so a uniform was definitely part of it, also all the smells. Mainly, I wanted patients to experience what I had during those times in the sick bay – a very clever person who cared for me. At first, I wanted to be a children's nurse and applied to many leading hospitals in London, including Great Ormond Street and Bart's. In those days you had to provide a photograph, which I did, and details of your father's occupation, which I left blank as I didn't know him at the time. I never heard back from any of them, even though I had seven relevant GCE 'O' levels.

The medical officer at the clinic where I was working as a school nurse assistant could not believe I had not heard back from any of these hospitals. He suggested I try his alma mater, St Mary's Paddington, but I was unfamiliar with that area of London and without Google to help in those days, I accidentally ended up at Paddington General. It was a happy mistake – I was quite delighted to be there and had three years of wonderful training.

What were the highs and lows of being a nursing student when you trained?

The highs were some of the subjects – I loved medical nursing, adored it. In those days many lectures were given by doctors and there was one registrar whose lectures I really enjoyed. He saw something in me and later said that he would help me if I wanted to change from nursing to medicine, but I was happy with what I was doing and never regretted it.

The other thing was the camaraderie of being in a small cohort – there were only 12 of us.

But I didn't like rules, I wanted freedom and so after

the mandatory year of living in the nurses' home, three friends and I moved out at the first opportunity and into a rented flat.

Another high was working on the wards and nursing older people. I loved listening to their stories, so I set myself a challenge of finding out as much as I possibly could about each patient. There was one particular experience where I spoke to an older woman and I was shocked at the life she had had, so interesting. Previously I had just seen a dependent older woman, but when I spent time with her, a tremendous sense of humour emerged. It was a good lesson for me.

Where was your first job after qualifying?
I stayed on as a staff nurse on the adult medical ward at Paddington for six months.

How did it compare with your expectations?
I absolutely loved it, adored it, but I had the idea that I wanted to do midwifery, the only real reason being that it was the done thing; you worked for a while as a staff nurse and then did your midwifery qualification.

How did your career develop post-qualification?
I went to Edinburgh to do my midwifery course at the Simpson Memorial Maternity Hospital, a very elite institution. The students were lovely, but while I was there the film *The Prime of Miss Jean Brodie* came out and I recognised her character in some of the tutors. I had a free spirit and liked to question authority. I wouldn't take things as given, and that became quite difficult. As a result of unfair treatment by a particular ward sister, I suffered a bout of depression and wanted to make a change. Institutions were not the right environment for me. By this

time I knew I wanted to be a health visitor. The matron was very good and said that she would give me a reference.

Partly to improve my French and to get away from the hospital, I went to work with a family in a suburb of Paris, teaching their children English – not an *au pair*, more a part of the family. They were both doctors who ran an obstetric clinic and it was just what I needed to get some adventure. But Paris was expensive – exciting, but I couldn't afford to do the things I wanted to do. When I told my employers, they said they didn't want to lose me and offered me the option of working in the clinic to earn more money. So from feeling quite poor I was suddenly very flush!

I stayed nine months and then came back to take my health visiting certificate at Chiswick Polytechnic.

Around this time, as a result of researching my full background, I found my father in London and the following year went to visit Nigeria for the first time. It bowled me over. I remember the warmth of the country and the warmth of the people and I really wanted to go and work there. My father was now living there and he sat me down and said: "Look, Elizabeth, I'm really pleased you want to come, but you can't come at the level you are, you would not be able to cope. You could come if you got to a more senior level because people would respect your authority and it wouldn't matter that you didn't know how to work in such different ways." That was the first real career counselling I ever had.

At that time, I was doing a certain amount of teaching and thoroughly enjoying it, but it seemed like a big step between that and a proper tutor's course. My father questioned why I couldn't do it straight away and so I did, becoming a community nurse tutor in 1975. After that I realised I needed a degree if I was going to go to Nigeria at a senior level, so a series of events led me to the advanced diploma in nursing studies in Manchester, and eventually a PhD in health education at the University of London's Institute of Education. My thesis looked at the experience of parents of children with sickle cell in Brent.

After 10 years as head of Brent Sickle & Thalassaemia Counselling Centre, I moved to the Institute of Child Health at University College London as a lecturer in community genetic counselling within the Mother Care Unit of Clinical Genetics & Fetal Medicine. In 1997 I moved following my appointment as Dean of the School of Nursing Studies, Wolfson Institute of Health Studies, Thames Valley University (now the University of West London).

In March 1998, a Chair in Nursing was conferred by the University and in September 1999 I set up and became Head of the Mary Seacole Centre for Nursing Practice in the Faculty of Health and Human Sciences. From 2004-2008 I was also honorary professor at the London School of Hygiene and Tropical Medicine. In 2001, I was made a Commander of the British Empire for services to nursing in the Queen's Birthday Honours, and a Fellow of the Royal College of Nursing in 2004.

Who have been the most important role models during your career? What qualities did you most admire in them?
Some of the ward sisters were important to me – I just thought they were fantastic people. Of course, there was the nun who nursed me as a child, but I was also impressed by some of the people in the residential school clinic where I worked as an assistant – two in particular. There was one younger woman and an older woman. They were so different, but I don't remember a single negative incident happening with either of them. The young woman was ultra-efficient and the older one very warm, so different

styles but both really good nurses. The headmaster there was also inspiring, particularly in the way he related to children with disabilities. The principal tutor during my training combined a no-nonsense approach with a good sense of humour.

What have been the biggest challenges for you as a nurse?
The practicalities of nursing – I could be quite cack-handed at times. I loved the academic side and the work with patients, but I wasn't always the best at the practical side of it. I so admired theatre nurses who made sure that everything was just so, it wouldn't have been for me. Another negative has been people who don't like being questioned and resent you wanting to know more, the hierarchy and kowtowing to medics. I love working in a team and I understand that there are different roles, but I don't understand people being subordinate.

Did you ever feel that the demands of the job put you under unacceptably high levels of stress?
At times yes, particularly when I moved to new environments. Although I am adventurous, I don't like a lot of changes. Getting to know the culture and rituals of a place can be challenging.

How did you deal with that?
I learned to be assertive, polite but assertive. I wouldn't get into an argument for the sake of it, but there would come a point where I could become argumentative. I used humour wherever possible. Usually people understood that I was asking for genuine reasons, but questioning practice did lead to difficulty in my health visitor placement. I questioned why data was being collected about patients

from the new Commonwealth and discovered that even people in the team didn't know. As a result my practice supervisor failed me and the college were stunned because I was one of their star pupils, so I took this to the medical officer of health and he investigated. He contacted the college and they called a meeting and I sat outside while they debated my future. Fortunately I passed.

What strategies did you use to get you through the most challenging times in your career?
Reading helped me a lot, music and friends. I was quite shy, having had a pretty sheltered existence, so the social side was difficult, but I had good friends who took me under their wing. I had to learn to open up to friends, though, that has been really important, as has relaxation and diet. And sleep! It probably helps that I don't drink and I don't smoke. I have also known when to leave a situation. If it is really too difficult, you have to have an ability to step back and to realise that other things are more important.

What are you most proud of in terms of your career as a nurse?
The sickle cell work. I am really proud of being part of setting up the first nurse-led sickle cell and thalassaemia counselling and screening service. And, probably inadvertently, being part of raising the profile of Mary Seacole and the statue appeal.

How has being a nurse affected other areas of your life such as family and friendships?
Nursing has dominated my life. As a single parent I had to fit my nursing around my daughter and my daughter

around my nursing, so that was how she knew me. Many of my friends are nurses and the irony now is that my daughter is an actress, Azuka Oforka, playing a nurse in *Casualty*, the BBC television programme. She is very proud of nurses in the NHS.

What would you say are the main qualities needed to be a good nurse?
You have to have curiosity about health and illness and how you can alleviate, prevent or reduce illness. If things go wrong, to have the courage to question the delivery of care and to own up if you have made mistakes. And it helps if you have the ability to see the limitations of everything.

In your opinion, how has nursing changed since you were starting out?
Certainly education and the experience of being a student has changed very much, compared with my own experience of a small cohort. Later in my career, I saw things from the other side, as an academic. While I can see the advantages of the changes in education that have taken place, I can also understand why students don't have the same sense of belonging to an NHS trust - everything is too big. When I started there was something about belonging. Certainly in the big universities today, especially in London, there may not be a sense of community. Size can be a problem, whether it is the university department or the NHS trust. Do students feel lost sometimes in the system? But the bonus is the ability to stretch students' capacity for self-learning, and the resources they have are mind blowing. However, I do have some sympathy with people who worry that to be a nurse, it may seem that you have to be very, very clever. I hope the progression routes stay there and that people are given the opportunity to

work towards the qualifications they need.

Would you recommend nursing to anyone considering a career in the profession today?
Oh, definitely. I'm very proud to be a nurse.

Key facts: Elizabeth Anionwu

When did you train as a nurse?
1965-68
Where?
Paddington General Hospital
Qualifications
State Registered Nurse, Health Visitor, Community Nurse Tutor, Advanced Diploma in Nursing Studies, PhD in Health Education
Current role
Emeritus Professor of Nursing, University of West London. Vice Chair, Mary Seacole Memorial Statue Appeal

Chapter Two

Protecting yourself from emotions around you

Every working day you will be dealing with people who are experiencing different levels of anxiety. Depending on where you work, this can mean regularly supporting people who are in a high state of emotion, often negative and painful emotion. In this chapter we look at how you can communicate well while maintaining your own balance and mental integrity.

I sometimes ask my nurse clients: "Do you realise how weird your working life is?" Usually they do a double-take, for them it all seems normal, routine, sometimes even boring and pretty much like everyone else's working day.

This isn't surprising. We all get used to what we know and it is almost automatic to assume that what we experience is pretty much what everyone else goes through. On top of that, health care is a bit of a closed world. Many people who work in healthcare come from whole families with a tradition of working in the caring professions. Frequently nurses' partners are other nurses and often social circles are made up of other health workers. So it all gets to look as if everyone lives this way, dealing with death, pain, fear and life-changing events as a daily occurrence at work.

You nurses are very competent, the initial selection process is tough, training is extensive and intensive and you are tested regularly. 'What's that got to do with anything?' you may be asking. Well, here is an interesting fact which you probably do not know, but which can affect how you feel about what you do: there is good evidence that people who are competent underestimate how good they are at their work. Conversely, people who are incompetent often overestimate their skills.

This phenomenon is called the Dunning-Kruger effect. Although it sounds paradoxical, it is logical if you think about it. People who are incompetent don't know enough to analyse what they do in a critical or reflective way so they can overestimate their performance. Those who are skilled, knowledgeable and competent know what they don't know so are consequently more aware of any shortcomings.

That can be a positive, you know your weaker areas and enjoy finding out more to update your knowledge. But it can also be a negative, you know your weak spots and you beat yourself up about them. Beating yourself up is never going to add to your happiness, indeed it will do exactly the opposite.

The 'high-end fashion store' thought experiment

So you are working in highly emotionally charged surroundings, taking great responsibility and may underestimate how good you are. Not a recipe for a stress-free work life, is it?

As I said at the beginning, this is unusual; most people do not live their work lives like this. Most daily working lives are very different and are conducted at a much lower emotional temperature.

I sometimes ask my nurse clients to do this quick thought experiment to prove this to themselves.

Imagine yourself working in a high-end fashion store as a sales assistant or a sales manager.

There you are at the start of your working day, in the softly-lit, elegantly-designed shop, wearing your designer clothes and ready for the next eight hours.

Who do you see and talk to? Who are you going to be interacting with between now and when you go home?

What do they expect from you? Close your eyes and imagine who is going to come through the door of your shop.

Let's see, first to come in is the woman buying the most expensive dress of her life for her daughter's wedding. Next comes the wealthy tourist on her twice-yearly visit to the UK to stock up on her wardrobe. Mid-morning, you have to deal with a cross person who cannot squeeze into a size 14, but is not going to admit it. She says it is your fault because your sizing is wrong. You have been well trained to deal with this sort of thing so you smooth it over and avoid a complaint.

After lunch comes a regular visitor; the fashion-savvy, but less well-off young woman who is trend spotting prior to seeing what she can pick up on eBay. Then a man comes in looking for a present for his wife but he has no clue at all about what she likes. And so it goes on, your feet might be a bit sore from the killer heels you have to wear to keep up the image, but apart from that it's all pretty straightforward. You don't really have to worry about who comes through the door.

All your customers are having fun, even for the fashion-serious their trip to your shop is not the most important thing in their life, or even in their week. Even the 14-plus lady will get over it; she has probably forgotten about it already. It's light, it's fun and not that serious. It's part of the fluff of life.

How many people do you think work in such

environments? I can't tell you how many work in the sort of posh shop we have been thinking about, but over four million people in the UK work in retail, that's compared to about 400,000 nurses working in the NHS.

So we can hazard a guess: there are more people going to work every day who deal with the light fluffy side of life than those who have to confront a lot of heavy emotions in their day-to-day work.

The importance of doing something important
You may have had a bit of a 'shall I change jobs?' moment when thinking about the posh shop, or you may have thought 'that's boring' or a bit of both, because of course you are well aware that there is a positive side to dealing with people at their most stressed and vulnerable.

It is important. What you do matters and can make a difference to those you are caring for now and in the future. People will remember the nurse who comforted them in the crisis. I remember when my Dad died – thanks Sarah, I can still remember that hug and you telling me how much everyone on the ward had liked him.

People are much less likely to remember who sold them a dress or a pair of trainers. The emotionally heavy work can give a deep meaning and a real feeling of fulfilment, which, as we have already seen in the last chapter, can be the route to true happiness. Working in an emotionally caring role creates the profound job satisfaction that many of you will get from your average working day. Probably, you went into the profession because you wanted to deal with the big issues of life rather than the fluff.

But sometimes, especially if you do not have access to good support and supervision, working in this environment can become overwhelming. We will talk about what happens when things get too much and you are in danger of burnout in a later chapter. I want to try to prevent you ever getting to that stage.

In this chapter I want to suggest some everyday, easy steps you can take to protect yourself and optimise your performance in the highly-charged circumstances in which you work.

Reframing your own thoughts and feelings

It is very easy, when faced with the emotional pain of others to mirror their feelings and thoughts. This can end up being exhausting and often counter-productive. People working in a professional caring relationship can fall into this emotional habit because they do not want to appear, or to be, distant or cold and because they value the empathy they bring to their nursing.

On the other side of the caring relationship, people who are sick and afraid can behave in certain characteristic ways. They often project magical powers onto those around them who they perceive as more powerful or knowledgeable than themselves, and, guess what, that can often be you. If you just absorb all these emotions, it can be a quick route to feeling inadequate and even guilty because you cannot make everything right.

So take a step back and decide what you can do in this encounter. Ask yourself what you can achieve realistically, what would you feel proud of doing? Then look at the situation and acknowledge any negative emotions or thoughts you are having. It might help to give these thoughts and feelings a name.

So, for example you may be faced with a relative who is angry because their loved one does not seem to be getting better. You do not know why their pace of recovery is slow and this is making you feel nervous about confronting the relative and defensive because you do not have the answers they are seeking. Acknowledge your own thoughts, perhaps they are: "I don't know why and I can't find out, the relative will think I'm incompetent". Perhaps you will call this feeling: "Oh no. What do I do?"

Now think of what is going on and how you can tell a different story with the same facts. Perhaps you can say to yourself: "I am looking after this patient to the best of my ability and I know he is receiving good medical intervention – people are different and I cannot change the rate of recovery. I do understand how worried the relative is; perhaps I can reassure them and that will help but if it does not, I can still say I did my best." You will find that adjusting your story begins to set up different and more positive feelings. You will feel more confident and relaxed. Does a name or phrase come to your mind? Perhaps you could call this state "Okay. Give support and explanation".

The second feels better than the first doesn't it? Even just thinking about the comparisons before you do anything shows this to you.

This is good in itself; you deserve to be able to do your job with positive feelings and positive feelings are good in themselves. You may also find that your changed demeanour makes it easier for you to achieve a better outcome for the people you are dealing with. If you are showing that inner confidence and belief in your own competence, people around you are more likely to trust that you are doing everything possible.

This is a great mindset to get into and you will find that with practise it can become second nature. But do remember that you can't win in every situation.

So if you sometimes fail to help people out of their negative emotional cycle, accept it. Do not use it as evidence of failure. Sometimes you can do everything right and it still turns out wrong. That's life!

How to say no

When people are frightened or feeling out of control they are likely to make impossible demands. Fear can force people into narrow and magical thinking patterns where they can become fixated with obtaining something which they have convinced themselves will solve all their problems. Aside from this, you may be faced with patients who have unrealistic expectations of what you can do. They may expect you to be able to sort out their social problems or access a new treatment they have read about on the Internet, for example. A few patients or relatives like this in a day can leave you feeling drained and isolated.

Learning some techniques to soften refusals can help. A good place to start is to acknowledge that refusal hurts – it's amazing how this can calm an angry or upset person. You can break their magical thinking state by turning the focus to the limitations of the real world. Phrases such as: "That would be good if that could happen but it can't because of . . . I know that is disappointing." "I know you really wanted 'yyy' to happen, but it is not possible because of 'xxx'."

The explanation here is important as it puts the person making the demands on you into an adult position where you are treating them with the respect afforded to an intelligent person who recognises how the world works.

Once you have done this you are in a much better position to put the focus on what you *can* do or what might help. Again this can help break the 'magical thinking' state. You can gently change the patient's focus from the one thing they believe will solve the problem to realistic alternatives. This might take some time and it does not always work, but it can help show that you are putting creative effort into coming up with a new solution.

Feel grounded in your professional knowledge and expertise and be prepared to share this. Do not be afraid to say you will not do something if your professional judgement is that it would be wrong to do so.

In acting this way, you are taking responsibility and showing your patient that you are using a wealth of knowledge and experience to help them. This may be painful for the patient and some will never accept what you are saying, but you stand a much better chance of entering into a positive dialogue about what you will do and then reaching an agreement or contract with the patient if you start with this mindset. You will cut down on pointless arguments, a benefit to both you and your patients.

Remember that a patient in the 'magical thinking' trap is feeling powerless and is unconsciously putting themselves in the psychological space or role of a powerless child. You, the one with the power, are put into the role of the all-powerful parent. This may involve conceptualising you as kind and wise or as mean and punishing, but it will always involve putting you in a role which assumes you have a power and influence which you do not. This can be very stressful and upsetting. It puts you in the uncomfortable position of being asked to deliver (and this can be as much about emotions as material goods) things which are just not possible.

People under stress are more likely to be angry and disputatious. If your patient is in the 'magical thinking' loop where they believe that if only the magical thing 'yyy' happened all would be well, they will be disposed to argue while they still believe there is any chance of getting this magical thing.

One way of breaking this loop is to say: "I will not do that" (because it is against all my professional knowledge) rather than: "I cannot do that'" (because of the rules, what my superiors say, for example). If the patient hears 'cannot' then they will often just move their thinking to the next level of the hierarchy or the next organisation where they might get a different answer. If the patient hears 'I will not' (because my professional judgement is. . .) then the magical loop is often broken and the discussion can continue on a much more adult-to-adult level.

An informal contract or agreement with a patient or relative about what each of you can expect from the other can help. It is an effective way to protect yourself emotionally as it means you can deal with problems and situations as they arise, measure what an outcome was and then move on. You will find it easier to deal with that horrible situation where you have so many things going on at once that you are spending all your time worrying about how to prioritise rather than dealing with the actual issues. It also allows you to reflect at the end of the day on whether you have achieved your outcomes and if there is anything to learn from where you have not.

***Case study:

Catherine says 'no'***

Catherine, a newly qualified staff nurse, described herself as being frightened of a patient who was aggressive and was demanding to be transferred to another ward, 'where the nurses treat you like a human being'.

Catherine felt that the patient was becoming increasingly angry and distressed and she was worried about the patient's wellbeing. She was also aware of the toll this behaviour was taking on herself. Catherine described waking up at night with the patient's voice in her head and not being able to get back to sleep.

I taught Catherine the 'sphere technique' (you can find it at the end of this chapter) to help her protect herself. Then we rehearsed how she could deal with the situation. Catherine felt uncomfortable saying 'no', so I asked her to write down 20 instances, in both her personal and work life, where saying no was the right thing to do. When she came back the next week she said this exercise had made her 'feel different' about the word 'no'.

We then went through what, in Catherine's opinion, the best outcome for her patient would be and Catherine practised saying calmly and clearly why it was best for her to stay on this ward. Catherine practised time-limiting the conversation and making it clear that the purpose was to explain the professional decision and how it was in the patient's best interest. She found that her new attitude meant the patient became less aggressive, and seemed happier. Catherine felt she had achieved considerable progress.

***

The benefits of setting an agenda

You can sometimes gain confidence in dealing with difficult situations if you plan well and then set an agenda with the relevant people. Begin by deciding what you want to or need to do in a particular encounter with a patient or client or their relative. Run through this in your head (or write it down if necessary) and estimate roughly how long it will take (if you do this regularly, you will find your time estimates become spot on after a while).

Be clear and honest about how much time you have to give to this discussion and deal with emotions up front as you talk together. If things are going very well you can reach an overt agreement on what you are each aiming to get out of this encounter. Overwhelming emotions can make it difficult to achieve a good outcome as the emotional load can stop the patient or client asking for the help, information or support they need. You can save time and get past the emotional blocks by asking direct questions such as:

- What is worrying you most about this situation?
- How are you handling the feelings around that?
- Is that working or do you feel you need more help?

Make your questions direct and bounded (one thing at a time) and allow the patient a chance to reply in the way they feel is appropriate.

Communication styles

If you are assertive, transparent and clear, you will protect yourself well and reach good outcomes for those you care for. The most important thing to learn is how to communicate in a way that will achieve the outcomes you want as an expert professional faced with a challenging situation.

Remember you cannot *fail* to communicate; everything you do is communicating something so why not make sure it is communicating what you want?

Non-verbal communication

We have all heard it claimed that most communication is non-verbal. Well, it is only sort of true; here are the relevant facts.

Some of the groundbreaking studies by Albert Mehrabian in the late 1960s and early 1970s found that 38 percent of all communication is tone of voice, and 55 percent is physiology (body language such as facial expressions, body movement, gestures, eye contact, touch, voice and body space) *in certain circumstances*. That *in certain circumstances* is important and key to understanding how we communicate. Mehrabian's formula has become something of a popular myth, but if you think about it for a moment, you will probably reach the conclusion that it is nonsense.

Try this thought experiment. Imagine standing in front of a friend with the intention of telling them, without using words, that you are going to apply for a new job, but you are worried about the interview and are not sure about the travelling distance if you did get it. It doesn't work does it? Or, as the old joke goes: if words only mattered for 7 percent of our communication, then no-one would ever have to learn Hungarian.

Poor old Albert Mehrabian has spent much of his career having to explain that the popular formula associated with him wasn't what he said.

His original experiments were based on communications about feelings and attitudes and he is very clear that these findings do not apply to other types of communications. Later research into verbal and non-verbal communication has found that when the receiver of the communication needs to judge whether it is true and how important the information is then verbal communication becomes very important indeed.

Yet Mehrabian has made some crucial discoveries. His real insights come in relation to the importance of congruence between verbal and non-verbal communication. He found that if our appearance, body language and voice tone are not congruent with our words then confusion and even distress can arise.

If someone is already at a low ebb this can lead to upset and even anger. So getting the non-verbal and verbal working together is especially important in emotionally-charged situations – which is where, as a nurse, you spend much of your working life.

So what is going on? The key thing is the way our brains process information.

The brain processes images much faster than it processes words and because of this, non-verbal communication is important as its message gets to the brain first. Added to that, when people are distressed they can find it difficult to take in words at all. So if your non-verbal signs are saying: "I'm rushed and anxious" and your words are saying: "relax everything is going to be fine" then the non-verbal signal will be picked up first and most strongly. It may even crowd out the words entirely.

Life will be easier for you and better for your patients if all the communication channels are working together. You might find this checklist helps your life run smoother:

• **How you look** Keep neat when you can, it is calming; it makes it look as if you are in control.

• **Your stance** Be relaxed and open. Don't fold your arms. Let your shoulders drop so your upper body looks relaxed.

• **Your voice** Breathe properly, if you are rushing around and you sound breathless you will come across as anxious and that will provoke anxiety in the person you are speaking to. Relax your throat by dropping your head to your chest, then swallow – this will help you control the pitch of your voice and stop you sounding squeaky (squeaky says scared and robs you of authority, so you don't want that).

I know I keep saying this, but it is so important I am repeating it: you cannot fail to communicate, so it's worth choosing to do it well.

Just as you cannot fail to communicate, neither can your patients. Even if a client is having difficulty verbalising, they will be telling you all sorts of things about themselves, if you have the skills to read them. Non-verbal clues can help you recognise your client's communication style. Most of us will use all these styles, but usually we favour one and use it most.

The main types are visual, auditory, kinaesthetic, and auditory-digital.

For example, some people will be primarily visual and often use phrases such as 'I see'. They will tend to speak quite fast and at a higher pitch. They will move their hands a lot. People who are mainly auditory will tend to have lower voices and will often talk to themselves or move their lips when they are reading. They will say things like 'that rings a bell', 'I hear that'. Kinaesthetic people do things slowly and breathe deeply, they have deep voices and will often stand near to those they are talking to or lean over them. They will use phrases such as 'I want to get a handle on this'. Lastly there are auditory-digital people who place a high value on logic and detail. They will use terms like 'that makes sense'.

Getting a feel for how people communicate can make your work smoother in two ways. Firstly, you can identify and deal with something that can be a source of annoyance. Someone with a very different system to yours can make you feel irritable. This is not because the other person is doing anything wrong, it is just that they are different.

I am auditory-digital and sometimes kinaesthetic persons, pausing before they speak and getting into my body space, make me uncomfortable. I probably come across as cold and snappy to them, especially if I am under pressure or not feeling at my best. Neither of us is wrong or right, we are just different, and since I recognised this I get much less irritable. This really is a case where a little knowledge can make a big difference. Once you begin to appreciate these differences you can value them. Also remember that none of us is purely one of these systems, we are all a mixture. So when you are with someone different, you can bring out that side of your personality. It can be done; I can now truly say that some of my best friends are kinaesthetics.

Secondly, you can tailor the way you send messages to

meet your clients' preferences. If you pick up that they are using one system, then replicate it in the phrases you use. They will quickly feel that the two of you are bonding and building a good rapport. They will like and trust you.

This is not as difficult as you might think; we do a lot of this instinctively as we all desire to get along with others most of the time. And as a nurse, you will almost certainly have very good instincts when it comes to relating to others, or you would not have become a nurse in the first place.

Mirror, mirror

We've just been speaking about language, let's bring in body language now and see how that helps too. Replicating the behaviour of those around you is as important with body language as with speech patterns. It's called matching and mirroring.

Next time you are in a pub or a restaurant look around you and notice how people are sitting. The people who look happiest, the people who seem to be getting along with each other and having a really good time will often be making the same type of gestures, sitting in the same posture and changing their posture and gestures at the same time.

This is something we do unconsciously all the time. It is a way of establishing rapport with those around us and saying: 'we are like you and we like you'.

The technique of using this natural behaviour has been refined and codified in the discipline of neuro linguistic programming (NLP). It is based on the established fact that when people get along they tend to use the same voice tone, phrasing in speech and body language. You can develop this innate skill to smooth the way in any situation where things might be tense or communication difficult.

There is a difference between matching and mirroring. A good description of the difference is given by Roger Ellerton. In his book *NLP Techniques that Anyone Can Use,* he explains: "Mirroring is as if you were looking into a mirror. To *mirror* a person who has raised his right hand, you would raise your left hand (i.e. mirror image). To *match* this same person, you would raise your right-hand (doing exactly the same as the other person). Some practitioners see a time difference between mirroring and matching. For example, if someone makes hand gestures while they are speaking, you would wait until it was your turn to speak before making similar (matching) hand gestures."

Successful matching and mirroring requires practice and also sensitivity – if done badly it looks like poor acting. Remember it is a technique which is just a conscious application of something we all do unconsciously all the time. So trust your instincts.

You can also use the opposite of matching and mirroring to diffuse difficult situations.

Here is how it works. If a patient is angry or distressed, then you do not want to mirror or match them, it will just raise the emotional temperature and it will also upset you, as our gestures and body language affect our mood. Instead you can change the mood by consciously using a different tone and stance. So, for example, if you are dealing with an angry or agitated person they will probably be speaking in a high, fast voice and fidgeting. So consciously lower your own voice and slow down your speech, and make sure your posture is still and relaxed.

Most people who go into nursing know a lot of this instinctively, the profession tends to attract good communicators who are sensitive to the messages others are sending out and use a natural empathy in working out how to respond. Taking that unconscious knowledge and refining and developing it, can help you protect yourself.

I want to finish this chapter by showing you a technique to protect you through your working day. If you are ever feeling bullied or pressurised this can help. It's a good idea to record yourself reading it. Keep it on your phone and then take 10 minutes to listen to it before you start work if you know you have an especially difficult day ahead.

Help yourself: the sphere

Make sure you are somewhere safe and secure where you will not be disturbed. Sit in a comfortable chair. Begin by breathing slowly and deeply. Put your feet flat on the floor and your hands beside you or on your thighs.

Then try to imagine as strongly as possible. Imagine you are in a wide open meadow and you can see for a long way. Look ahead of you and you see a shape in the distance – it is surrounded by a glowing golden light. You are curious about the shape and begin to approach it. You are somehow attracted to this light, you know it is safe and powerful and good.

As you walk towards the shape it becomes bigger and clearer. You feel that this shape is here to help, you feel drawn towards it – you know it will protect you.

As you get closer you see that the shape is the shape of a sphere. It is transparent or maybe translucent. It may be clear or perhaps it has a gentle colour. As you approach you see the sphere is just a bit taller than you; you walk around it and notice a door in the side.

You step inside the sphere and feel a sense of safety and

warmth infusing you. You feel relaxed and secure and strong.
Focus on your breathing and notice that the sphere moves in time with your breathing. It is under your control. Imagine you stretch out your arms and the sphere stretches with you. Play with how the sphere responds to your breathing and your stretching.

Now imagine things you don't like and see how the sphere can protect you. It is strong and anything you don't like cannot get inside. Imagine anger, hurts, shouting just bouncing off the sphere while you stay calm and safe inside.

The sphere is there to always protect you. Your sphere is invisible to others. Only you know it is there and it can be with you whenever you need it. Now decide how you will use the sphere. Decide how you want to keep it with you to protect you from now on.

You choose how and where you will keep your protective sphere.Perhaps you will make it very small and keep it in your pocket. It can be taken out and grow like an inflatable tent whenever you need it. Or perhaps you will keep it in a secret place knowing that when you call it will come rolling towards you to help you.

Choose what is right for you and keep your sphere in its safe place. When you are faced with a difficult situation secretly activate your sphere and keep yourself safe and calm.

***

Stories from a nursing life: Fiona Murphy

"I am always happier talking than writing"

Fiona Murphy's commitment to listening to those she

is caring for and acting on what they are telling her

has always been at the centre of her nursing

philosophy. This ability to see things through other

people's eyes led her to make revolutionary changes

in bereavement care.

When did you decide to become a nurse?
From the age of about three. My parents bought me a
uniform for Christmas and they had to force me to take it
off so that they could wash it.

What was the appeal?
I suppose I am a fixer. I really wanted to work with people,
it is just in me. Also, my dad died from a heart attack when
I was 18 and my mum was only 42. I wanted to find out for
my mum exactly why my dad had died. I needed to
understand what had happened to him.

Was it your first career or did you do something else first?
Between leaving school and starting my training I worked
as an auxiliary nurse in older people's care and that
convinced me that nursing was the right thing.

Did you consider any other careers? If so, what were they and why did you reject them?
I never considered anything else.

How did you decide which branch of nursing to go into?
I wanted to work in an intensive care unit partly because my father had died in ICU and that gave me a specialist interest in cardiac ICU.

Did you have an image or fantasy about what nursing would be like?
I was not an academic achiever – I knew I was a compassionate person and so I thought I would suit nursing really well.

What were the highs and lows of being a nursing student when you trained?
I was very stressed about the academic side of things, basic theory, which is why I took the 2-year enrolled nurse training; more practical. But the high was qualifying – I loved it, such a sense of achievement. I am competitive and I want to be the best I can be, so qualifying was brilliant.

Where was your first job after qualifying?
Intensive care at Harefield Hospital in Middlesex.

How did it compare with your expectations?
I had an overwhelming need to understand how my father had died. Working in a specialist cardiology ICU was like a light bulb going on.

How did your career develop post qualification?
Conversion from EN to RGN brought promotion from a D Grade (under the old clinical grading system) to an E grade.

As a cardiac nurse specialist, I became a junior ward sister and then moved to Stoke Mandeville hospital spinal injuries unit for six months to broaden my range of skills. From there I moved to Lancashire with my husband and two children because the children were starting school and I knew that was where I wanted to settle; that was home. I became a junior ward sister at Bolton ICU and took my English National Board qualification as an ICU generalist, ENB 100. Working part-time with two children, I went for a sister's post and then moved up through F to G grade and finally in January 2002, an H grade post working as donor liaison nurse. That was when my remit exploded and I was given the target of increasing organ donation in a 6-bed ICU. It was an incredibly steep learning curve.

After six months of working with the traditional donor model, known as the Spanish model, I had another light bulb moment, thanks to a man called Harry whose wife died in ICU during the summer of 2002. She was on the donor register. They had been married for 50 years, had no children, no other family, and his wife had collapsed suddenly while she was out walking the dog. He wanted to cuddle her and so I left him with her for a while and then I helped him wash her, even though this would normally be the nurse's role. He did not want her organs to be donated because he felt that she had suffered enough. I realised then that if he had agreed to donation, he would have been followed up and offered all kinds of support. But without agreeing to donation, he got nothing. So I decided that I would follow up with Harry.

This difference in approach to bereaved relatives based on organ donation became a bit of an obsession and eventually I went to the Chief Executive and said that I couldn't do the job under the existing policy. He supported me to stay as donor liaison nurse but with a wider remit to cover bereavement. I put together a team of three and together we implemented a new bereavement policy, not just in ICU but across the whole hospital. Complaints fell and in fact donor rates went up considerably as I somehow hoped and believed they would. The service started to win awards – from the *Health Service Journal*, *Nursing Times* and NHS North West Innovations.

Then, in 2011, I became the *Nursing Standard* Nurse of the Year and the publicity brought national recognition for the service. Previously, there had been no link between palliative care, bereavement and organ donation, but we brought them all together and it worked. I was then seconded to Salford to lead on implementing the same changes we had introduced at Bolton.

After that I went to Wigan with a similar remit and in 2012 we linked everyone together and I became Assistant Director of Nursing with responsibility across all the trusts.

Who have been the most important role models during your career? What qualities did you most admire in them?

As a nursing auxiliary, before starting my training, I learned so much from a matron called Valerie Chowdhury. She was everything that I wanted to be – just brilliant with patients, so focused and even though she could be a firm taskmaster, she was consistently kind and reassuring with patients. She was the most important role model for me. I have never forgotten her.

What have been the biggest challenges for you as a nurse?

The biggest challenge for me has been, without a doubt, the academic side of things, particularly writing essays. I have been driven by a desire to know more, to study theory and academic research because I have wanted to use that knowledge to develop services, but it has not been easy. I am a great networker, I know I am a good clinician, I can and have presented at international conferences, but I am always happier talking than writing. Self belief was also an issue for me; I'm not ashamed to admit that. It's something I have had to work on.

How have you dealt with a high stress environment?
Everybody says it is hard to work in this environment because you see the worst of everything, particularly if you are in a crisis role. But I truly believe it is a privilege to be with people in these last moments, or with relatives and friends. Peer support has been very important for me and clinical supervision is a vital opportunity to share experiences. Always working as a team, involving people, listening and sharing have made it easy for me.

What are you most proud of in terms of your career as a nurse?
The innovations we have made and the way that has improved the whole experience for the bereaved. Really it is about making an obvious difference to people's lives. Most of my family were academic achievers and I really wasn't, but my grandmother used to say: 'don't worry, she'll make someone a lovely wife'. I am so proud that nursing has led to many, many professional achievements.

How has being a nurse affected other areas of your life such as family and friendships?
My husband, Peter, is also a nurse so it is very much a part of who we are as a family.

What would you say are the main qualities needed to be a good nurse?
Kindness and compassion. If you don't have that then this is not the job for you.

In your opinion, how has nursing changed since you were starting out?
I keep hearing that we don't have time to care because of poor staffing levels. If I'm honest, I don't really believe that is true. You have to be able to respect patients' dignity, to provide good care and to value what we do, whatever the circumstances.

Would you recommend nursing to anyone considering a career in the profession today?
Absolutely. My son, Ben, has just qualified and is working in intensive care, so he must have understood how much we loved our job.

Key facts: Fiona Murphy

When did you train as a nurse?
1987-1989
Where?
The Whittington Hospital in North London
Qualifications
Enrolled Nurse; RGN after conversion course; Postgraduate diploma in death, bereavement and donation studies
Current role
Assistant Director of Nursing, Bereavement & Donor Support, Salford, Bolton & Wigan NHS Foundation Trusts

Chapter Three

Recognising burnout and how to stop it

Burnout is a wholly negative state where you feel

overwhelmed by the demands of the job. People who

give of themselves in emotionally charged

environments are especially at risk.

Everyone says they are burnt out these days. From city bankers to professional athletes, the idea that we all hit a brick wall has become common currency. It is true there have been many changes to working lives which may be bad for our health. For example, many of us are working longer hours and new technology is leading to a rapid blurring of the lines between work and home. Everyone in work is experiencing these changes and is at risk. But within this generally risky environment it may be that people in the caring professions, such as nurses, are in particular danger.

There is a good reason for this; to do the job well means engaging your own emotions in your work. The very thing which makes nursing such a fulfilling job, that one-to-one contact with other people when they are vulnerable and needy, can also be the thing which leads to feelings and emotions so overwhelming and uncomfortable that you may feel you can no longer cope. If you are heading towards burnout you will be stressed, but you can be stressed without being burnt out. In fact, stress is not necessarily a negative factor.

A certain amount of stress can be useful to motivate and drive you, to get you going for the   challenges of the day ahead. This type of stress is often characterised by engagement and active emotions. Here is an example from a client of mine.

Case Study Sue steps up

Sue had just been promoted to a more senior role on a new ward. She remembers a day when she was very busy on the ward (unusual that!), but this was also the day when she recognised that a young medic, on the ward for the first time, was out of his depth and she supported him.

She chatted to him and said how it could be a baptism of fire and re-assured him that he would get used to it. She also gave him some practical advice about how to question a very elderly patient. She felt stressed about this, it was her new ward and she felt her responsibility very strongly, but she was concerned about possibly crossing professional boundaries and running up against a notoriously bad-tempered medical consultant.

When I asked her to describe how she felt, she described feeling tense and being aware of a tightness in her chest and of her breathing being faster than usual.

She said she felt 'a bit nervous' but she also said she felt very 'clear and focused'. Afterwards she felt confident that she had handled what could have been a very awkward and potentially dangerous situation well. She felt good professionally because she had offered the practical advice which had ensured the best care for her patient and she had also supported a colleague, which produced a different sort of good feeling.

As I listened to her recalling this, I was noticing a lot of very positive things. She was animated and active and using lots of action words; saying she had been working with all systems firing, that she was sparky and full of life and it made her feel good to be going beyond the routine and outside of what had been her comfort zone. She felt herself growing into her new, more responsible role, or to use her phrase 'stretching up'.

Yes, she had felt 'a bit nervous' but she recognised that it can be good to be nervous when you are confronting new experiences and you need to learn fast and to act quickly. She had also had a very useful insight: good stress is not a permanent state. She had been stressed about one event which, through her own expertise, action and efforts, she had dealt with successfully. Then it was finished and she could go back to what she described as her 'normal work head'.

***

How too much stress can lead to burnout
What my client Sue described is an ideal way to experience stress and use it for a positive purpose – in these cases stress enables you to perform as well as you can under unusual pressure and then return to your own 'normal work head'. (It's not just your head by the way, all your body systems

return to normal in this healthy cycle).

Unfortunately, for many of you nurses the work situation can be one of constant pressure and competing demands which you do not have the time or perhaps the support and skills to fulfil. Being constantly over-busy and never having time to do anything well is not the road to go down. It leads to unhealthy stress that is overwhelming, constant and never-ending. This can lead to burnout.

Burnout is a wholly negative state, characterised by feelings of disengagement, loss of motivation, feeling powerless and helpless in your professional life. Worse than that, if it goes on too long it can even spill over into your wider life, of which more later. The signs of burnout can be both mental and physical. They include exhaustion, loss of appetite for healthy foods, lowered immunity and a feeling of hopelessness. If you are experiencing burnout you will find it harder and harder to relate well to your patients and colleagues.

How to recognise signs of burnout
One of the problems with burnout is that by the time you are at risk you are not in the best situation to recognise the signs. So it is worth knowing the types of behaviours and feelings which could be a warning. This is by no means a complete list, but if you are experiencing any of these or anything similar then you could be heading for trouble.

• One thing to watch out for is the 'one size fits all' approach – if you are treating all your patients the same without noticing how their different personalities mean they react differently, then it may be time to think about whether you are experiencing burnout.

• Another sign can be falling back on procedures and rules in an overly-prescriptive way, doing things by the book because your creative powers to adapt the procedures to fit the patient are feeling to difficult for you at the moment.

● Downplaying a patient's feelings and emotions can be another indication of approaching burnout, if you find yourself believing that a lot of your patients are making a fuss or being unreasonable, that can be a warning of trouble.

● Removing yourself emotionally from the illness and pain your patients are experiencing can also be a warning. If you notice you are spending more time than you know you need to on tasks which take you away from patients, or if you are volunteering for jobs which take you away from face-to-face contact then you may be heading for trouble. You are developing a coping mechanism here, but it may be one which is unacceptable to your colleagues, unsustainable for you and bad for your long-term career prospects. And if you came into the profession because you love helping people it can mean you lose that joy and fulfilment which is such a part of nursing.

Expectations and reality

Christina Maslach and Michael Leiter have done lots of work on burnout in organisations. They have surveyed over 10,000 people and reached the conclusion that burnout is caused by a mismatch between expectations and reality in six areas. These are:

● the amount of work expected of you
● how much control and decision-making power you have
● rewards, both material and acknowledgement of your role
● a good community where you are respected and supported
● a fair and transparent environment
● a workplace which shares your ethical values

Based on this, they came up with this quick assessment tool to determine if you are burnt out or at risk of becoming burnt out.

You can see the assessment tool on the next page. It is

of most use if, rather than just answering 'yes' or 'no' you nuance your responses a bit. Before you respond to each question consider whether everything is just right, whether it is a bit mismatched or whether it is very mismatched.

If everything is just right then well done, you have chosen just the right job for you and everything is going well, long may it continue. Most people can tolerate a few mismatches and to be honest most of us have to, especially in times of cuts and re-organisations. If, however, you have a lot of mismatches then you are in serious danger of burnout and you need to take action. Another point to consider is how important each of these factors are to your personal value system and way of operating. For example, if you are a very social person then even a bit of a mismatch in the community section might upset you greatly, whereas if you are more introverted and happy to be independent then you will tolerate this. So take account of your personality and what is important to you as you ponder the questions.

Workload
- The amount of work to complete in a day.
- The frequency of surprising, unexpected events.

Control
- My participation in decisions that affect my work.
- The quality of leadership from upper management.

Reward
- Recognition for achievements from my supervisor.
- Opportunities for bonuses or raises.

Community
- The frequency of supportive interactions at work.
- The closeness of personal friendships at work.

Fairness
- Management's dedication to giving everyone equal consideration.

○ Clear and open procedures for allocating rewards and promotions.

Values

○ The potential of my work to contribute to the larger community.

○ My confidence that the organisation's mission is meaningful.

If you find you have mismatches in quite a few areas then first of all you can breathe a sigh of relief and congratulate yourself. This may sound an odd thing to say as you are probably feeling rotten and even anxious about the future. But now you have made an important step in recognising that you have a problem, what that problem is and in what areas it is most severe. These are the first steps to doing something about it.

It may sound trite to say that, but one of the horrible things about burnout is that it can make you feel trapped. For a start, it is usually accompanied by feelings of exhaustion, loss of confidence and lack of motivation. Not an ideal state in which to contemplate change is it?

On top of that if you are burnt out because of your work environment then there is a good chance that at least some of your colleagues are heading the same way. It is very likely that you are experiencing difficult, short-tempered or morose colleagues in an over-stretched environment. That doesn't sound like a fun place to work every day. As our mums always told us, misery loves misery.

So it's miserable isn't it? Yes it is, but not insurmountable.

Do anything. Yes anything!

After all this gloom there is some good news. You will feel a bit better if you do anything, and I mean anything. I bet you don't believe me, so let me explain what is behind this thinking. One thing absolutely central to burnout is feeling a lack of control. If you can take back control, even in a very limited way, you are telling yourself, both consciously and unconsciously, that there is a solution, another way. A little bit of progress can bring a big reward.

It's worth remembering that most of our behaviour, our feelings, emotions and moods are formed outside of our conscious control. Once you are in a negative way of thinking, whatever the cause, it can be difficult to know how to break it. If you are burnt out, or heading that way, the misery and unhappiness can seem overwhelming. Don't despair, there is a way out. Unhelpful thinking is a habit, and like all bad habits it can be broken. It might be a struggle sometimes but it can be done.

Here is something you can do straight away. It is a classic in the field of positive thinking, and is a simple tool which works. It is usually called 'The 3 blessings or 3 good things'. This was developed by Dr Martin Seligman who we have already met as one of the major developers of positive psychology. He argues that, for sound evolutionary reasons, we have a predisposition to focus on events which go wrong in our lives rather than what goes well, (the evolutionary reason being that for most of the history of our species a bad hunting day or mistaking a fierce animal for a friend could be the difference between life and death, so dwelling on these mistakes and mishaps and learning how to avoid them in the future made sense).

So we have this inbuilt pessimism, this habit of gloom, and it has its benefits, it enables us to learn lessons and avoid repeating dangerous mistakes. But this way of thinking has a big disadvantage as well; by concentrating on the negatives in our lives we can get into mental habits which lead to anxiety, depression and burnout.

Dr Seligman has conducted research over many years which has shown that increasing positive emotion using targeted mind exercises has long-term benefits. One of the exercises he developed is known as the '3 blessings' or the 'what went well' exercise. This is a way of encouraging ourselves to get into the mentally healthier habit of focusing on what goes well, then enjoying that by remembering and re-experiencing it and then taking credit for it. Many therapists, coaches and psychologists have used and adapted this simple, evidenced-based tool. Here is a version which I use with my clients. Seligman stresses the importance of writing as well as thinking in this exercise. So prepare to write. A few of you might really hate writing, if you feel very strongly about this you can do this exercise using audio, or even video recordings. The important thing is that you record your thoughts, which will send a message to your unconscious that this is important. It also means you can track progress over time.

If you decide to write, buy yourself a good quality notebook. Don't go for the supermarket budget version. Go to a proper stationery shop and choose something you really like. While you're there buy a decent pen as well. If it suits you, choose coloured ink, your favourite colour. This will make your writing feel very different from the note-taking you do at work.

Start by taking ten minutes for yourself at the end of the day. Make sure you are by yourself; it is good to tell your loved ones you need these few moments to yourself. It's not that long; everyone can fit in ten minutes. Choose a time near to your normal bed time (if you are working shifts then make some time between coming home and going to bed) as the exercise works much better if you sleep on it.

Create a nice atmosphere for yourself; sit somewhere comfortable and pleasant, which will make you feel better before you even start. Take your lovely notebook and pen, notice how holding the pen feels and run your fingers over the paper, feeling how smooth it is under your fingers. Deliberately breathe more slowly, this will relax you and help you focus.

Now you can start to write down 3 things which have gone well for you today. It doesn't matter how small they are. It could be that you had a good laugh with a colleague at handover, or you noticed a lovely sunset when you left work, or a patient gave you special thanks as they left hospital. Perhaps your heart leapt when you picked up your little boy from nursery or your partner gave you a special hug when you walked in the door. There will always be three small pleasures, even in the worst day. Of course this might have been a day when you met the love of your life, or your new nephew was born. It's good to write the big things down as well.

There may be days when you really believe nothing good has happened at all, those truly awful days we all have from time to time.

If you have had a day like this, remember it doesn't matter how small the good things are. You're alive, you ate today, your kids are okay and healthy and one did well in a test today, and . . . get the idea? There are always some things, so write down your 3 good things for today.

Okay, next step. What is causing those good things to happen? Are you doing something to cause them to happen? I bet you don't think about this very often. Most of us just let the world carry on its merry way, without taking time to take credit for our role in creating the swirl of stuff constantly happening around us. But most things that happen to you happen, to some extent at least, because of what you do.

Now you have your 3 things, begin to think about why they happened. Some things seem to just happen. . .that lovely sunset as you left work for example. . .and that's good, it's good to notice that the universe around you is wonderful.

But you did something too didn't you?

You had to notice that sunset. You've probably left work on other days and the sky has looked just as good, but you didn't see it. So why did that good thing, that lovely sunset happen to you today? Perhaps because you were so positive and attuned to your environment that you took time to notice the good things in nature around you? This might be the cause or there might be a different reason for you. There is no right or wrong here, what you come up with is your reason and it is valid and right for you.

Sometimes it will be obvious that your 3 things happened because of what you did or who you are. That patient saying "thanks love" happened because you are a good nurse didn't it? And you can bet that patient is now telling her family and friends how great you were. Your heart leaping when you see your child?

That is because you are a good parent and your child is happy and pleased to see you because of your parenting. What do you do that makes you such a great parent? It can be useful here to think about the little things, perhaps these are habits you are not even conscious of, they have become ingrained in your everyday life. What are they? How do you do that? How do you make that happen? Then there will be the good things which have happened to other people which give you that boost. Think about what you can learn from these things. Is there something in there that you could do too?

Write down the causes of your 3 good things and why your good things happened to you. This might feel a bit awkward at first, we are often too modest and not in the habit of taking credit for our achievements, but try it and you will be amazed at the results.

Do this every day for six months. It will change your thinking habits. You will also have an extensive record of your

3 good things in your lovely notebook. Take some time to look back whenever you feel like it, well done!

Help yourself: 3 good things

A) Take your best notebook and good pen

B) Find somewhere quiet and tell everyone not to

disturb you for 10 minutes

C) Write down 3 things which made you feel good

today

D) Write down what you did to help them happen

***

Goal setting

Another way you can protect yourself against burnout is to set yourself some clear goals. Notice the words, 'set yourself' here. These are not targets from your manager or hospital or clinic. These are about you getting the most out of your working life. Setting goals is about expectations, what you expect from life and what other people can expect from you.

It is also about setting boundaries, so you make sure there are clear areas of your life which are for you and in your control. Having goals in place will enable you to test out how things are going for you. Make them realistic and achievable and have a clear idea about what you need to do to reach your goal. Set yourself a timescale in which to achieve them.

If you are concerned about burnout, there are two areas which are especially important: making the most of time away from work, and making space in your workday so you are not going at 100 per cent for the whole time.

Start by setting a goal of taking time off. A good starting goal is getting a bit more time for yourself completely away from work. That's not going to work, you say, I'm always much too busy. Well here is an interesting fact. Organisations working in disaster areas have recognised that even in the most dire and pressurised circumstances their workers need some clear time off. The Red Cross, for example, now aims to give workers a day off every week, even when they are working in a crisis situation.

So set yourself a goal of some clear time for you. If you are stuck in a mindset where you really believe you have no time at all, start small. Aim for just a couple of hours a week and build from there.

So what are you going to do with this time? Perhaps you have a burning desire to do something, a hobby or a challenge, which you have longed for but never thought possible. If that is true for you then plan to do that thing now. For most of us, however, it can be hard to think of what to do, especially if you are out of the habit of taking time for yourself.

So, once again, start small. You do not want to pile unnecessary pressure on yourself at this stage. Exercise can be very good. Increasing evidence is showing us just how good exercise is mentally and physically. But one word of warning. If you feel you might be approaching burnout it is important to be gentle and gradual. Choose something that is going to help you and that you know you will enjoy. Don't pile extra pressure on yourself. The challenges and pressure of, say, running a marathon or taking on a team sport can be exhilarating, but if you are feeling in danger of burnout you need to be careful that you are not transporting a tendency (common in burnout) for frenetic work activity into your non-work life.

It is often better to start with something easy, gentle and short; remember your rule is taking away pressure not piling it on. Anything which you find relaxing will do (and if that really is extreme sport then fine, you can ignore everything I have just said). If you feel comfortable doing something physical then that is probably the best choice as you will be getting all the positive benefits of exercise as well. So try walking, jogging, yoga, whatever you fancy. If you don't like physical exercise this may not be the time to start as it could end up feeling like just another chore. Instead try some mindfulness exercises or some relaxing self-hypnosis instead (go to www.nursesbook.com for examples).

Making space in your workday
Nurses work harder and under more pressure than most people; the role often demands that you answer the needs of others rather than schedule your own time. This makes making space a real challenge and sometimes it just isn't possible, but there may be more you can do than you think.

Start off by identifying what is robbing you of your time. You may notice that these are tasks which are below your skill level or add nothing to what you see as the key purpose of your job. Do not be afraid to delegate if this is feasible.

Ask if it is possible to stop doing the pointless tasks, discuss this with your colleagues, you may occasionally find that this task does have a use and then it will not feel so bad doing it, or everyone may agree it has no purpose so you can discuss how to create the process necessary to stop doing it.

The next step is to prioritise as much as you can. You probably try to do this and sometimes, even most times, it falls apart. It will not always be possible to prioritise because of pressure of work, but it could be going wrong because of what you are doing. Prioritising relies on three other things being in place. You need to: be able to set goals clearly; know how to delegate; have the skills necessary to say no.

Let's look at these in order. To set goals clearly use this check; what would happen if you didn't do that thing you say is the number one goal for the day? If it wouldn't matter that much then consider that it might not actually be today's 'must do'. Delegation is essential within your professional and legal responsibilities. Remember people often like being asked, just make sure you ask in a respectful and inclusive way, stressing that you have other things which must take priority for the good of the whole enterprise. Make it clear that you trust your colleague to do the task and you will support them and ensure that they have your backing should they need it.

If you find it difficult to delegate then it may help to find a role model. If there is someone you know who does this very well then watch them, listen to how they speak, watch their body language. Look around to identify people who could take on some of these delegated activities. Who would blossom by being asked, within the bounds of your professional responsibilities and knowledge set? Choose the person who will most appreciate being asked.

Saying no is something which comes from a calm and positive assertiveness. You are more likely to say no, and get a smile in return, if you indicate that you may be able to help later. So say something like: "I have to do this first, but come back to me later if you still need help." Or: "I have to leave on time today, so I can't fit it in I'm afraid, perhaps we can get together to sort out how we fit this in later in the week?"

Another technique which can soften the blow is to set your refusal in the context of what you are there for, what you do in the team and as a team. So saying something like: "Sorry, I can't do that because I must finish xxx and we did agree that was a priority for this team because yyy depends on it." Try to come up with alternatives if you can. "No, I can't help with that but try John, he is a real expert and will do it three times quicker than me anyway."

Of course, people asking for your help can be doing so for all sorts of reasons. If someone is out of their depth, perhaps because they do not have the skills to carry out their role, then take a step back and decide what you can do about this in the longer term.

Then there are those people who are difficult and/or lazy and are always trying to get out of doing things. Here, a more direct approach helps. Smile as you refuse, it is very disarming. You might say: "I know you can do that better than me, it's much more your area." A little flattery can go a long way: "You are much better qualified to handle that, you'll get a much better outcome than me." Lastly, don't be bullied by the difficult types; sometimes a straight, simple no is what you need: "I can't manage that I'm afraid." Try it, after the first time it is not as scary as it seems.

Stories from a nursing life: Laura Downes

"We nurses remain friends forever"

Laura Downes always wanted to be a nurse and has loved every minute of it. She has also found the courage to make a mid-career change to journalism, but still keeps her nursing values at the centre of her life.

When did you decide to become a nurse?
I never considered anything else.

What was the appeal?
Nurturing I guess. I loved dolls. . .I was a very girly girl. I didn't know it at the time, or can't remember, but apparently my Mum always wanted to be a nurse and was forbidden by her mother, my Grandmother. Incidentally, when I left office work to become a student nurse my grandmother, who I loved dearly, refused to have anything to do with me for at least a year because she believed that nursing was immoral!

How did you take the decision - alone, with help from friends, family or a careers adviser?
Mainly alone as I remember. I suddenly took the decision one Sunday to go through the Yellow Pages and send off letters of application to *all* the local hospitals. I had

enormous support from my parents, who were thrilled. The careers adviser at school was awful as I was leaving aged 16 and you had to be 18 to start nursing. I insisted I wanted nursing and also asked about cadet nursing but she kept trying to push me into going into banking, which was ludicrous as I was terrible on numbers! It was as if she was on commission.

Was it your first career or did you do something else first?
From the age of 16-18 I worked in admin for the NHS. I did this to get as near to nursing as I could and to get as much insight as possible. I wasn't hospital-based. I was in a very high management office and I was the lowest of the low, but loved it and was treated well and supported to go on to nurse.

Did you consider any other careers? If so, what were they and why did you reject them?
No not really. However, I've always said that my second choice would have been a career as an English teacher, so maybe that's a yes? I dismissed it as my school grades were so poor.

How did you decide which branch of nursing to go into?
To be honest, in the '70s things were so different I don't think I even knew about anything other than adult general nursing, so that's what I applied for.

Did you have an image or fantasy about what nursing would be like?
Oh yes. . .and all I imagined became a reality, as in happy, sad, hard work, wrinkly people, messy stuff, exciting, rewarding etc.

What were the highs and lows of being a nursing student when you trained?
Too many to tell! But overall, it was so happy. Highs were:
- Leaving home at 18 and being independent
- The enormous bond (which continues today) with several other nurses/flatmates
- Continual learning and support from other nurses/tutors/students
- Diversity and change (every three months) from things like geriatrics/mental health/A&E/midwifery/surgery etc.
- The uniform! I took pride (we all did) in the uniform, including hats, belts and cloaks
- The fun. We had so much fun. Imagine being at RCN Congress for a 3-year period, it was along those lines
- The pride in being a nurse
- The love received from patients and relatives
- Making a difference – getting people well and seeing them home home safe and well

And the lows were:
- At times, exhaustion. This included finishing a shift at 9-9.30pm then going back to get changed, joining others for a drink (not every night) and getting up at 5.30am to pin hair up under hat and be back on shift at 7am
- Grief and shock and sadness. My first death was a lady I found dead in bed on day 9 into my training. My knees shook!
- Lack of money – at times this was worrying – I ate a lot of jacket potatoes having taken the rotten bits off
- This might sound daft but the cleaners who cleaned our homes! They used to assemble to chat and make coffee and at times brought their children in while we were trying to sleep. There were often arguments
- Dragging yourself into work even when you felt really ill but too scared to go sick

Where was your first job after qualifying?
Medical Staff Nurse at my hospital – a popular post with many other applicants but I was selected.
How did it compare with your expectations?
Fantastic! Loved it. I stayed there for a year before I transferred to A&E and only moved to gain further experience. I loved mentoring and the responsibility of running a ward.

How did your career develop post qualification?
- 1979-80 (1 year) medical staff nurse
- 1980-82 (2.5 years) A&E staff nurse (senior staff nurse for last 6 months)
- 1982-84 maternity leave
- 1984-85 agency nurse briefly then I was a bank nurse back at my old A&E (running the department on and off)
- 1985 Matron of an independent nursing home and registered manager with social services – overseeing building development and employment of staff, development of policies and assessment and integration of clients, while pregnant again. At the end of 1985, my second son was born – I worked up until the day before I had him and was back two weeks later for brief visits
- 1986-1991 Practice Nurse
- 1990-97 Group Editor at Publishing Initiatives, a small publishing company
- 1997-2015 RCN Publishing Continuing Professional Development Editor and then Clinical Editor and Special Projects Manager, finally Group Educational Development Editor

Who have been the most important role models during your career? What qualities did you most admire in them?

No pioneers but strong leaders. My role models in nursing have always been those I worked very closely with. Oddly, they were mostly the strict 'matron type' sisters I worked with and, although they could be scary, I always knew they cared, not just for the patients but for us as nursing students also. Linda Thomas and Jean Gray in my publishing career. I learnt so many things, such as not to panic when in fear, to look outside out of the box and find alternative solutions.

What have been the biggest challenges for you as a nurse?
To challenge attitudes, particularly as a young nurse. You're either an 'angel' or a 'saint' or a pushover. I feel so strongly about this.
Every nurse in the '70s and '80s carried a reputation as 'easy'. I cannot describe how many awful moments I had because of that. . .bear in mind my grandmother's attitude too!
Other challenges were the strict regime and that you never answered back, even if innocent, the shifts, days to nights, but I accepted that as part of the job.
Oh. . .and the pay I guess!

Did you ever feel that the demands of the job put you under unacceptably high levels of stress?
No. It's part of the job and what you sign up to. I'm not saying it wasn't stressful, and there was lots of unpaid overtime, but like I say. . .

If so, how did you deal with that? If not, how did you manage to avoid this in such a high stress environment?
Talking it through when you get home, with family or (nursing) friends.

What strategies did you use to get you through the most challenging times in your career?
As above. I never had to consult a professional.

What are you most proud of in terms of your career as a nurse?
So many things. . . I was great at diagnosis, over and above doctors at times. As a practice nurse, I persevered with a patient I knew was very ill, although I didn't know quite what with. The patient was losing patience with me and despite referral to a local consultant he sent her back to me with a curt note as in 'nothing wrong'. I continued and saved her life insisting on further blood tests, she was instantly admitted to ITU and survived. It was a matter of days before she would have died. I was known for recognising unusual symptoms in A&E and the doctors always listened to me and trusted my gut instinct.
I'm so very proud to have moved from hands-on nursing to journalism. I still feel like a nurse and have loved doing things for nurses. I never knew I had it in me to make such a big career change, but have loved every moment and all the challenges involved.

How has being a nurse affected other areas of your life such as family and friendships?
Neighbours, friends, friends of friends, family, friends of my children etc, etc see me as 'on call' permanently for advice/dressings/triage. It's fine though, I love it! The only other thing I guess is that we nurses remain friends forever, whereas other people in other careers lose touch.

What would you say are the main qualities needed to be a good nurse?
Compassion. Empathy. Respect. Regard. Stamina.

In your opinion, how has nursing changed since you were starting out?
I learnt more in my time from sitting on the bed, holding the patient's hand and listening than I ever did from books, theory and management. Both nurses and patients (and their carers) would benefit from more time together. There's too much top-down management.

Would you recommend nursing to anyone considering a career in the profession today?
Absolutely!

Key facts: Laura Downes

When did you train as a nurse?
1976-1979

Where?
Queen Mary's Hospital, Sidcup, Kent

Qualifications
1979 Registered General Nurse (RGN)
1990 BSc 2:1 (Hons) in Psychology, Open University

Current (or most recent) role
Group Educational Projects Manager, RCNi, formerly RCN Publishing

the nurses' handbook

Chapter Four
The challenge of shift work and how to cope

Working shifts is an inevitable part of nursing, it is bad for our health but some people are more able to tolerate it than others. The picture is complex and the more we understand what shift work does to the body, the more ways we are finding to protect ourselves.

Over a quarter of NHS staff are working regularly between the hours of 7am and 7pm and many non-NHS staff will also work at nights. Night working has been the subject of much research and many policy statements, a sign in itself that there is cause for concern. In this chapter, I will look at the pros and cons of shift work, and suggest some ways you can maintain your wellbeing when you are working outside of the standard 9 to 5.

There are various settings where you may work shifts. As well as the biggies: accident and emergency nursing and working the night shift on general wards there are also emergency mental health nursing teams working at night, or you could be offering 24-hour telephone advice, working one-to-one in a patient's home or be in charge of a care home. And that's just for starters.

Working at night is part of the job for many nurses and it

brings its own benefits and challenges. Some of you may love doing the night shift. Many nurses working in a hospital setting on the wards at night say it gives them more freedom as there are fewer managers around and they can make more decisions for themselves. Some of you also say that there is a special feeling in night-shift teams, the more relaxed atmosphere and being at work when most people are not, means night-shift teams often bond more strongly , something that those of you who particularly value working in strong, close teams will appreciate.

The quieter atmosphere, with fewer regular tasks and procedures being carried out, means night shift nurses often find they have extra time with patients; most patients are asleep so nurses have time to give more one-to-one attention to those who are awake. Nurses with introverted personalities, who like working in a quieter atmosphere, may find that some night work is enjoyable for you, but of course not all night work is quiet.

Working in A&E at night offers a completely different experience, especially at weekends when units can be busier than on many daytime shifts. Some nurses find that the 'day for night' experience this gives can be exhilarating and they enjoy the fast pace and pressure to make quick decisions. A client of mine, who has worked night shifts on A&E by choice for years, says one of the best moments of her working time is walking to her car after the end of the night shift and enjoying the early morning. At this point she goes through a mental ritual of wishing all the patients she has seen throughout the shift well for their onward journeys whatever they may be.

So there can be positives to working at night, but there is another side to the story.

Many people who work nights find they are drowsy at work; they worry that they can't think straight or make good decisions. There has been a lot of research on health and shift work, both within the health professions and more widely, and most shows that shift work is not good for our health and well being. Overall, most studies show that shift work is bad for both nurses' health and their career patterns, with many studies from different countries showing that nurses working night shifts are more likely to have a poorer work-life balance and to experience less job satisfaction and career progression.

Then there are the health problems, with nurses who have worked nights for long periods showing higher levels of obesity, diabetes and hypertension. A large scale study which monitored 75,000 female registered nurses in the United States over 22 years (through the Nurses Health Study) found that nurses who worked for longer than six years doing rotating shifts suffered serious health consequences with higher levels of cardiovascular disease and some cancers. [1]

It appears that rotating shifts are especially bad for health although we don't yet fully understand why. Our knowledge is beginning to increase as researchers investigate the links between how different shift schedules (with varying durations and frequency of change) affect individuals.

Sleep patterns, Circadian rhythms and light
There is considerable evidence that shift work severely affects sleep patterns and this is very damaging to health and well being. An American survey by the US National Sleep Foundation in 2008 (The National Sleep Foundation Poll) found over a third of shift workers said they did not get enough sleep compared with just over a tenth of non-shift workers.[2]

The survey also found that one in ten shift workers suffer from serious sleep problems and other related issues. This has been called 'shift work disorder' and includes different problems related to sleep, such as excessive sleepiness in the day and insomnia at night as well as difficulty concentrating, irritability and depression. Disrupted sleeping patterns are a big cause of ill-health for shift workers, but they are not the only problem. The damage to health from shift work seems to have two main, and linked, causes. Firstly, there is our biological body clock, situated in the suprachiasmatic nucleus (SCN) in the hypothalamus. This generates the Circadian rhythms which regulate many of our body's physical processes and those processes determine important patterns of behaviour, such as body temperature, hunger, alertness and sleep. This biological mechanism is responsive to a whole number of external stimuli, but the most important one here is light.[3]

Working at night disrupts the body's Circadian rhythms and lowers levels of melatonin (due to lack of exposure to light). A study carried out in 2012 measured how well nurses and midwives working night shifts synthesised melatonin and came up with a preliminary conclusion that working eight or more night shifts in a month could disrupt this process.[4]

Shift work and social pressures
Separate but linked to this are the social pressures of shift work. All shift workers report disrupted eating and sleeping patterns. A recent report by the Health and Social Care Information Centre has shown that shift workers are much more likely to be overweight, have diabetes and suffer from back pain.

Yet the picture is not clear; some people tolerate shift work better than others, the reasons for this are complex, but we are getting to understand them better. A big literature review by the Sleep Medicine Review (of over 60 studies) attempted to identify what sort of people are okay with shift work. It found that young extrovert men who believed themselves to be in control of their lives tolerated it best. A study of nurses in a number of European countries in 2014 found that the worst health and career outcomes were among nurses who had no say in whether they could work shifts.[5]

Owls and larks

Another important factor was 'morningness', otherwise know as 'lark or owl syndrome'. It is known that younger people tend to be more 'owl' and most of us become more 'lark' as we age. German professor, Till Roenneberg has found a pattern where most children, who are larks, get more owl-like until they reach 20, then the process reverses. This basic pattern is very strong, but there are variations within it.

Neurogeneticist Dr Louis Ptacek has discovered some of these. He studies families with what he describes as 'familial advanced sleep phase syndrome' (people who come from families where everyone is up at 4am ready to go birdwatching or out on a hike) and found they had a mutated gene (a similar gene, if mutated in mice, made the Circadian 'clock' speed up), so it may be that there is a strong genetic base for our morning or evening preferences.

If you are a strong evening person you will find it easier to tolerate night shifts, or evening shifts. It is worth finding out where your natural preferences lie when you are thinking about your career choices.

You may find yourself doing different types of shifts and shift patterns within relatively short periods of time, particularly in the early part of your career. If this is happening to you it can be a good idea to keep a diary to track how you are feeling on the different types of shift patterns. You may tolerate some better than others and this is useful information to have when you make choices about your career.

***Help yourself:

are you a lark or an owl?***

Here is a short quiz, I give my clients to assess whether they are a lark or an owl.

If you were completely free to choose, when would you get up?

    a)   5-6.30
    b)   6.30-8.00
    c)   8.00-9.30
    d)   9.30-11.00

How do you feel after you have woken?

    a)   Fine, ready to go
    b)   Okay after a few minutes
    c)   I need a half hour to feel fully awake
    d)   I need at least an hour to feel fully awake

How hungry are you when you wake up

    a) Very
    b) A bit
    c) I want to eat about an hour after getting up
    d) I don't want to eat until much later

You have one really demanding, important task you need to do in your day. If it is entirely up to you what two-hour window would you choose?
    a) Early morning
    b) Early afternoon

c) Early evening
d) Late evening

A friend asks you to join a project between 10 and 11 at night; do you feel

a) I can't do that
b) Don't want to, but I like you
c) Okay
d) Great I'll be there

If you have to stay up later than normal would you

a) Wake up at the normal time next day
b) Wake up at the usual time and sleep later in the day
c) Wake up then go back to sleep
d) Not wake up until later

Do you use an alarm clock?

a) Never
b) If I have to get up very early
c) Yes I wake up on first ring
d) Yes I have to have it very loud and still take ages

If you were completely free to choose would you go to bed

a) At your usual time
b) An hour later
c) Two hours later
d) Much later than that

If you selected all 'As' you are an extreme lark and will probably be uncomfortable with shift work. If you selected all 'Ds' then you are an extreme owl and may find working nights is a pattern which is comfortable for you. If you are in the middle you will tolerate some shift work but a pattern of all or permanent nights may eventually get you down.

Coping with the physical effects of shift work
Of course being very tired can affect your driving ability, which is presumably why the Western Australian Government Office of Road Safety went to the trouble of putting together some very useful advice on how to look after yourself if you are working shifts. If you find yourself in a situation where you are having to change your shift patterns every few days (this is known as fast shift rotation) then they suggest:

• Try to spend some time in daylight before and after a night shift
• Try to sleep for a short time in the afternoon before the shift starts
• Eat lightly, but several times during the night shift

If you are changing shifts every week or so, they suggest:
• Go to bed as soon as you finish your night shift rather than waiting until later in the day to sleep (by that time your Circadian rhythms will be in full day mode and you will find it harder to sleep)
• Nap in the afternoon for no longer than 30 minutes if you still feel sleepy
• Try to avoid full daylight when you leave work after a night shift, for example wear sunglasses if you walk out into a bright summer day
• Try to eat regular meals, including a full 'lunch' throughout your night shift.
• On your last night shift adjust your body back to daytime by sleeping no more than three hours that

morning, and then getting a full night's sleep the next night
- On the days following your night shifts get as much exposure to natural daylight as possible; this will help your body return to a normal daytime setting.

Diet
Eating fresh, healthy foods and exercising will help. So good common sense looking after yourself will help you cope with shift work, whichever shifts you are working. There are some diet suggestions which are specific to shift work, however. Try to eat regular, light meals, choose easy to digest foods and avoid spicy and fatty foods. Avoid sugary foods as they will cause sugar spikes, which are particularly harmful when your natural balance is being upset by shift work anyway. You will also process sugar less efficiently at night so it is even more likely to increase your weight. Drink water regularly throughout your shift but tail off towards the end so you are not woken by a full bladder when you sleep after your shift.

Keeping alert at work
Many of the standard ways of keeping alert involve stimulation. These things seems to help: bright lights, noisy music, a cool temperature. Of course none of this is much help when you are trying to keep things quiet, dark, warm and peaceful for your patients!

If you can't open all the windows on the ward and get the music blasting, is there anything you can do? Here are some tips.

Take moderate exercise just before you start your shift. Spend just a few minutes in bright light as often as you can and take a short walk outside of your standard work environment. If it is possible get a full spectrum light somewhere in your work environment (you can get small visors, like a cap which you can just slip on for a few moments when you are out of public view) and expose yourself to it when you are feeling drowsy. This light will give your Circadian rhythms the message that it is day and time to work.

When you get home and are ready to sleep make sure you do the obvious, like shutting off the phone. It is also important to make your bedroom as dark as possible. Even if your eyes are closed, your brain will still register sunlight which is the most powerful way in which nature tells you to wake up. Invest in blackout curtains and blinds.

Finally, you will need to pay off your 'sleep debt'. Think of it this way, you will need one hour's sleep for every two hours awake. This does not change just because you are working at night, so when you come off night shift the first thing you need to do is pay your body back that sleep debt you owe, and as soon as possible. If you do this, you will recover more quickly and enjoy your time off.

A good routine is to sleep for a few hours when you get home, just to refresh yourself, then get up and go out to expose yourself to as much natural light as possible. As a bonus, take some gentle exercise to get your system functioning at a slightly higher level. Make sure you do something which you find mood-lifting, whether that is chatting to a friend or doing some gardening; it doesn't have to be anything spectacular, in fact it is better if it isn't as you want to keep things relaxed and gentle, but make sure it is something you enjoy. Be careful to avoid artificial stimulants in the course of this day, so don't drink coffee or alcohol as this will upset your sleep patterns later.

What you do next will depend on whether you are a lark or an owl. If you are a lark, try to go to bed a little earlier than you normally would on your first non-shift night. If you are an owl then plan to lie in a little later than you would normally.

Note the 'little' here. You need to reintroduce your normal sleep pattern gently, so perhaps go to bed an hour earlier or get up an hour later. You may find it difficult to sleep this first evening; if you do then try using a sleep app of gentle hypnosis or relaxing beats which induce your natural sleep patterns.

Getting to sleep

Hypnotherapy works very well for insomnia and you can visit a local practitioner or even buy an app for your phone. For many people, though, listening to their own voice works best. Below is a short script which you can record for yourself - put it on your phone and sleep well. You don't have to copy this exactly, treat it as a guide and put in any metaphors or words which you know you find especially relaxing. If you would prefer someone else's voice you can listen to me by downloading an audio file at www.nursesbook.com

The script uses all the senses and you can adapt that to your own ways. For example, you may be strongly led by one of the senses. If you are a very visual person, stress those bits, if audio then spend longer on the listening bits. Don't be afraid to experiment, you might want to record several versions and see which works best for you. Finally, don't worry if you fall asleep before the end!

Help Yourself Sleep

Read the script below, paying attention to the parts which seem most relevant to you. Rewrite any parts in any way you feel is helpful.

Talking yourself to sleep

I am enjoying the dark and the quiet, I am feeling the soft

sheets on my body, I can hear my own breathing. . .I focus on my breathing and breathe. . .more deeply. . .more slowly.
. . I focus on my feet and tense all the muscles starting with my toes my feet my ankles then I relax

I do this again
Then I tense my calves
And relax
Then I tense my thighs
And relax
Then I tense my core muscles
I relax
Then I tense my core muscles
I relax
Then I tense my core muscles
I relax
Then I tense my core muscles
I relax
My whole lower body feels heavy and relaxed; it is an effort to move.
I allow that feeling to move into my chest and my shoulders
Like a calm wave
I allow that feeling to move down my arms

To my elbows
Into my wrists
Into my fingers

First of all my thumbs completely relax, I couldn't move my thumbs even if I wanted to. Then my forefingers completely relax, I couldn't move my forefingers even if I wanted to, Then my middle fingers completely relax, I couldn't move my middle fingers even if I wanted to. Then my ring fingers completely relax, I couldn't move my ring fingers even if I wanted to. Then my little fingers completely relax, I couldn't move my little fingers even if I wanted to,

My hands feel warm and totally relaxed, that feeling moves up my arms and into my neck
My shoulders drop down into the bed
Now my face is relaxing
My tongue drops to the bottom of my mouth
My eyelids are so relaxed I couldn't open my eyes even if I wanted.
The very top of my head feels totally relaxed.
I focus on my breathing and notice how regular and calm it is.
I focus my mind on the colour I find most calming – secret just for me.
I think of all the words I know to do with sleep
Dreams
Slumber
Bedtime
Catnap
Dozes
Naps
Repose
Rest
Shuteye
Siesta
Forty winks

Keep going over that list adding new words as they appear
Now I can create sounds which remind me of sleep
I hear my breathing

Now I feel feelings connected with sleep

The sheets on my body
The support of the bed

I think of the words to do with sleep
Dreams
Slumber
Bedtime
Catnap
Dozes
Naps
Repose
Rest
Shuteye
Siesta
Forty winks

And I add some words if I want
I hear my breathing
Now I feel feelings connected with sleep
The sheets on my body
The support of the bed
I think of the words to do with sleep
Dreams
Slumber
Bedtime
Catnap
Dozes
Naps
Repose
Rest
Shuteye
Siesta
Forty winks
And I add some words if I want

I hear my breathing

Now I feel feelings connected with sleep
The sheets on my body

The support of the bed.

I now picture myself. Lying in bed. Snoozing and dozing. I
watch myself sleeping.

Imagine myself sleeping and dreaming. And drifting off. A
part of my mind is helping me relax. And I can imagine
waking, several hours from now, refreshed and happy.

References

1)
http://www.channing.harvard.edu/nhs/
2)
https://sleepfoundation.org/sleep-polls-data/sleep-in-america-poll/2008-sleep-performance-and-the-workplace
3)
https://www.nigms.nih.gov/Education/Pages/Factsheet_CircadianRhythms.aspx
4)
https://www.circadian.com/blog/item/44-adapting-to-shiftwork-5-influencing-factors.html?tmpl=component&print=1#.VdGBtflVhB
5)
http://www.ncbi.nlm.nih.gov/pmc/articles/PMC4196798/

the nurses' handbook

Stories from a nursing life: Jean White

"Not just one, but many careers"

Chief Nursing Officer for Wales, Jean White's nursing career has taken her from operating theatres in Wales to the heights of government and the European Commission. She has loved every moment of her journey.

When did you decide to become a nurse?
I had done very well academically up to GCSE O levels at 16, and I was head girl at both my secondary schools, private and public, so the expectation was that I would go on to university after A levels. However my A level grades were disappointing, mainly because I had become distracted and just did not work hard enough, there were so many more exciting things to do at that stage in life. While I later felt very guilty about this in terms of how much my parents had invested in my future, at that stage I rejected academia. My mother's best friend was a nurse and somehow it was listening to her stories that prompted the idea of taking a vocational rather than an academic route.

What was the appeal?
I realised that I wanted to work with people. I felt I needed

to apply myself vocationally, to do something that I could really engage with and that would make a difference to people's lives.

How did you take the decision - alone, with help from friends, family or a careers adviser?
There was very little time between my A level results in August and starting my nurse training in October, so it was quite a quick decision in the end, just a few weeks. My mother's friend thought I had many of the qualities needed to be a nurse and so she helped me arrive at that decision.

Was it your first career or did you do something else first?
I wasn't one of those little girls who always wanted to be a nurse. I do remember playing at being a nurse, as many children do, but nothing more than that. Over the years various ideas had come up, such as being a vet, but no one thing stuck.

Did you consider any other careers? If so, what were they and why did you reject them?
In many ways my decision to start nurse training was a rebellion against the academic pathway, ironic because it turned out that much of my working life has been spent as an academic, but at that stage I wasn't ready for that. In those days, pre-registration really was vocational training with very little academic input. I was under pressure from my mother in particular to take a decision and start working!

How did you decide which branch of nursing to go into?
When I qualified I was given a job at the Singleton Hospital in Swansea where I trained. I worked as a theatre nurse and really loved it.

Did you have an image or fantasy about what nursing would be like?
Not really. The short space between deciding what to do and then starting training meant I didn't have long to think about it.

What were the highs and lows of being a nursing student when you trained?
In terms of highs, it was very exciting, lots of new experiences, meeting and working with different types of people that I would never have come across before - and the things I was involved in for the first time: seeing a baby born was just amazing; in theatre watching surgery and wondering how on earth people could heal after such invasive procedures; laying out a body for the first time and being with people who were dying. It was and remains a real privilege to be with people when they are going through those experiences.

In terms of lows, it was not being allowed to speak up, the feeling that I had no voice. I asked questions about why we were doing things a certain way and I felt frustrated by the `because this is the way we do things here' response. I wanted to know what the evidence base was for many of the things that we did, but it seemed there was a local way of doing things and that was enough. It was never enough for me. I asked why and it is an approach that has stayed with me throughout my career.

How did your career develop post qualification?
I loved working in theatre. It meant being able to give full attention to one patient at a time, and I really enjoyed seeing the immediate results of the care I had given. The environment suited me. I got on very well and was given a

lot of responsibility. In order to further my expertise in that area of care I moved to London to take up the full time 12-month English National Board 176 Operating Department Nursing Certificate at the University College Hospital, before moving back to Wales where I held a number of posts as staff nurse and sister specialising in orthopaedic and trauma theatre nursing. I enjoyed the complexity of trauma and particularly loved passing on knowledge to students. This led to a teaching qualification in further education and a full-time post, first as a lecturer then as a senior lecturer in the School of Health Science at Swansea University.

At that time, I was one of only 11 female senior academics in the university. As well as teaching, I managed the registry functions of admissions and examinations for the school, and published in nursing journals. In 2000, a 6-week secondment at the Welsh National Board for Nursing, Midwifery and Health Visiting (WNB), an autonomous body set up by government to handle aspects of registration and to carry out quality assurance for education, turned into 6 years working in two national bodies. During this time I went from nurse advisor to director in the WNB and had to then close down the organisation as it was replaced by a new government organisation with a wider remit, Health Professions Wales (HPW). I joined HPW as nursing adviser and became director in 2004.

When this body was also closed following a government 'bonfire of the quangos', I joined the Welsh Assembly Government as a Nursing Officer, working to the Chief Nursing Officer (CNO), Rosemary Kennedy, advising on a wide range of important policy areas: nurse education, nurse regulation, regulation and development of healthcare support workers, non-medical prescribing, workforce modernisation, professional career development, care of the older person and protection of vulnerable adults.

When Rosemary retired, I acted up as CNO until being interviewed and appointed to the role substantively in October 2010. I recognised that it was a huge step change in responsibility as I became head of the nursing and midwifery professions in my country of birth. At the same time I knew it brought a lot of opportunity to influence the development of the professions as well as develop and implement health policy in Wales. I am by and large able to determine where I focus my attention while supporting the devolved government in Wales and it has given me great opportunities to contribute to the development of the nursing and midwifery professions, not just in Wales and the UK, but also internationally.

It is a demanding role, but as research shows, the more control you have over your working life, the less likely you are to suffer from harmful stress.

In addition to being the Chief Nursing Officer I am also Nurse Director of NHS Wales. This latter part of my job means I am responsible for the professional performance and development of Health Board/Trust Nurse Directors and the nursing and midwifery professions in NHS Wales. As CNO I contribute to the development, promotion and implementation of health and social care policy including working across the UK, Europe, internationally and with the World Health Organization. I contribute professional independent advice on nursing and midwifery to Welsh Government and contribute to the corporate management of NHS Wales. In addition, I am executive policy lead for:

- Maternity Services
- Patient Experience in health services
- Community Health Councils

- Child Safeguarding in NHS Wales
I share policy responsibility with the Chief Medical Officer for quality and safety in the NHS.

Members of my team provide the main health advice for people with learning disability in Welsh Government. I am currently the chair of the second phase of work to implement 'Strengthening the Commitment', which focuses on modernising learning disability nursing in UK and Eire.

The title of Honorary Visiting Professor to the School of Nursing and Midwifery Studies, Cardiff University was conferred on me in January 2011, and I was made Fellow of Swansea University in January 2013 with the honorary award of Doctor of Science. I was made Fellow of Bangor University in July 2014.

International work has always been an interest. I have undertaken work on behalf of the EU Commission as part of the assessment process to determine country readiness to accede to the European Union. I worked with the governments of Estonia, Slovenia and Czech Republic.

Following a three-month leadership placement in WHO (two months Geneva and one month Copenhagen) in 2009 I have regularly provided advice and support to the WHO European Office. In 2013 I was formally recognised as an expert nurse adviser to the WHO European Region. In July/August 2015 I worked in the Copenhagen Office to finalise the 'Strategic Direction for Nursing and Midwifery towards Health 2020' and developed a monitoring tool to track country progress in the 12 objectives it contains; and finalised the compendium of good nursing and midwifery practice roles within the region to share innovations in practice. These documents were launched at the Regional Committee of the WHO European Region in Vilnius, Lithuania in September 2015. I was honoured to be one of the speakers at this launch.

Who have been the most important role models during your career? What qualities did you most admire in them?
My parents were both incredibly hard working – my mother is 77 and still running a newsagents to this day. There was no tolerance of laziness when I was growing up and that has stayed with me, I abhor laziness, I would much rather people try and fail than not be bothered. Eve Sergeson was one of my nurse tutors and was a marvellous and inspirational teacher, who emphasised the importance of compassion in care. She and her colleagues made sure I began my nursing career with the patient firmly fixed at the core of all I did. It illustrates how important it is to get the initial education of nurses right. Lots of other people have helped and supported me throughout my career, but I wouldn't necessarily call them role models, although I will always be grateful to them.

What has been the biggest challenge for you as a nurse?
Wherever I have encountered situations in which the potential of nursing/midwifery and nurses/midwives is not recognised, for example the view by some that health professionals such as nurses don't need to have a degree-based initial education. That says to me that nurses are seen to be of lower value and status compared to other health professionals - that we don't need to use our brains at work, even when there is now a growing body of international evidence that points to improved patient outcomes and reduced mortality when nursing staff have graduate preparation.

Did you ever feel that the demands of the job put you under unacceptably high levels of stress?
There is a lot of stress in nursing, the environment can be stressful, but I like a degree of stress and much of it can be

positive and stimulating. After some years working as a senior lecturer (nursing) and head of registry at Swansea University, I was feeling burnt out, worn down. I was juggling what in hindsight were actually two jobs.

How did you deal with that?
With support from the head of school, I went on what was supposed to be a 6-week secondment with the Welsh National Board.

What strategies did you use to get you through the most challenging times in your career?
I have always been self-motivated, I don't like being bored, and so I have made changes when I needed to. I have been able to recognise when I need to step away.

My husband, Andrew, has been a tremendous support. We met when I was a staff nurse and he was a junior doctor, he has been my bedrock ever since.

What are you most proud of in terms of your career as a nurse?
There is a lot that I'm proud of. Having rejected academia as a teenager, I think the guilt of letting my parents down, and recognising all that they had sacrificed for my education, drove me on to achieve in the academic world. I am really proud of the recognition from universities – a Fellow of Swansea University where I used to work, and visiting professor at Cardiff. Getting my PhD was also a great moment for me.

In my government role, I think it would be achieving the government standards for advanced practice for health professionals in Wales, something that has not happened elsewhere. I am proud of the work I and my team are doing in ensuring safe nurse staffing levels in NHS Wales. I am also very proud of the work I do through the WHO internationally.

How has being a nurse affected other areas of your life such as family and friendships?
Being a nurse is part of who I am and I hope I am authentic with everyone I meet. People can be intimidated by the status that goes with the role of Chief Nursing Officer, but I don't think I put on airs. When I meet nurses and midwives I want to make sure I get as much from the encounter as possible and you have a richer discussion if everyone is at ease. I like to be part of a team. For example, it has been 9 years since I left Health Professions Wales, but the team still meets up on a regular basis for supper.

What would you say is the most important quality needed to be a good nurse?
More than anything, you need to care about other people, to understand that it is a privilege to do this work. That will come across in how you think and how you deal with people. You do also need to be bright and to expect a process of lifelong learning, striving all the time to be better at what you do. A sense of humour is a must.

In your opinion, how has nursing changed since you were starting out?
Nursing is now evidence-based and the status of the profession has definitely gone up. We have overcome the idea of nurses as doctors' hand maidens. Practitioners are now seen as educated professionals with a stronger voice. Huge numbers of nurses are prescribers and many are working as advanced practitioners.

Would you recommend nursing to anyone considering a career in the profession today?
Yes, absolutely. Nursing is not just one career but many careers which can take you into all sorts of different fields. Clinical practice offers opportunities in a variety of settings – hospitals, the community, public and private sectors, or the less obvious including working as an occupational health practitioner or even in the leisure industry. You can become a teacher or registrar, even a government adviser. There are few professions that offer so many opportunities.

Key facts: Jean White

When did you train as a nurse?
October 1979-October 1982

Where?
Swansea

Qualifications
State Registered Nurse; ENB 176 (Operating Department Nursing);Bachelor degree in Nursing; MSc in healthcare management; PhD; Postgraduate Certificate in Education (FE); Registered Nurse Teacher; Honorary Doctor of Science, Swansea University

Current role
Chief Nursing Officer for Wales/ Nurse Director NHS Wales

Chapter Five
Life moves on: how to get the best from change

As we go through life, changes happen and we can feel

a loss of control over events which affect our lives. How

can we exercise a measure of choice when we don't like

what is happening around us?

Most of the events we are told are stressful in life involve big changes. So is change itself the cause of stress? There is a lot of evidence that it is and that it can make us ill.

Back in the 1960s, psychiatrists Thomas Holmes and Richard Rahe developed a scale to assess whether stressful life events correlated with ill health (it is still used today and known as the SRRS scale).

Their answer, which has been borne out by many subsequent studies, found that they did. The most stressful life events are hardly surprising: death of a spouse, marital separation and imprisonment are the top three. But dismissal from work comes in at number eight and retirement at number ten. Business readjustment and change to a different line of work are in the top 20 stressful life events and in the top 30 come changes in working hours. Unsurprisingly, the scale shows that bad things are stressful, actually they are the most stressful, but change, even if it concerns developments which are presumed to be pleasant, can also be stressful. Vacations and 'outstanding personal achievements' also make it onto the scale. What is going on? Why on earth should going on holiday induce feelings in us which can be so damaging they can lead to illness? There is an argument that evolution has hard wired us to resist and avoid change. After all you never know what is around the corner, literally as well as metaphorically, so best to stick with what you know. Our brains recognise this and consequently change sets off the 'go on alert, fight or flight' response, which is both tiring and uncomfortable.

Processing change involves the higher level thinking centres of our pre frontal cortex. Using this part of our brain uses lots of energy so we try to use it sparingly and default to the familiar as soon as we can.

On top of that our brains make neural connections which reflect what we do regularly. Think of it as a path across a field, if you walk it every day it will become easier and wider and you will always follow that path.

It will feel very difficult and uncomfortable to set off across the long grass. Neuroscientists describe this process with the phrase: 'Neurons that fire together wire together'. With the development of brain scans we can see evidence that developing certain habits alters the very structure of the brain. For example, studies by Eleanor McGuire at London's University College found that London taxi drivers, who have to memorise tens of thousands of different routes, had a much larger hippocampus (the part of the brain which is used in navigation) than other people.

There is lots of evidence that we find change difficult. But of course we *do* change all the time. If we never changed, we would remain the same helpless baby we were on the day we were born and that doesn't work does it? Civilisation would never have got started!

Just stop to reflect and you will see that you are constantly undergoing the most massive changes. These happen fastest and most profoundly when we are very young. Think of how you changed between being born and the age of five, and when this was happening you didn't mind a bit, instead you welcomed it. Changing at this time is just a great big adventure. All children want to grow up don't they? Have you ever heard a child say I don't want to be six, I want to stay five?' If you did hear this, alarm bells would probably ring and you would see it as a sign that the child might be having some problems.

So when do we learn to fear change and why?

As well as the physiological reasons to do with our brains there are also social reasons. At around the age of eight we develop our sense of other people as independent from us and begin to realise we are not the centre of the universe. We can become acutely attuned to how others, and particularly those closest to us, are reacting. As part of this process, we pick up tensions from others, especially our parents. Often they will be displaying anxiety about changes happening to us, from changing school to the first date, to going on holiday on our own for the first time, to our first job. It's no wonder we receive the message, subconsciously, that change causes worry, therefore change must be dangerous and should be avoided.

Change is a demanding process. When we are making changes our whole system will be in a state of high alert. This is necessary because we need to have all our senses attuned to new situations, so that we can process them and decide what to do. This can be exhilarating, but it can also feel a bit frightening. It can also be tiring if it goes on too long, which is why constant change can be draining and stressful.

On the other hand, the best events of our lives also represent change.

If you are married, your wedding day represented quite a big change didn't it? But you probably enjoyed it. Going off to university, getting a new job, buying new clothes, getting a new haircut – all represent change, minor and major, and all can be fun.

So change presents a complex picture

There is, however, one sort of change which we mostly don't like and that is when change is forced upon us. Constant change is draining, especially when we cannot see the point of it. Big organisations, and health services are usually big organisations, are notorious for instituting constant change. And it is one of the main reasons people who work in health services say they are stressed. On top of this, badly managed change causes all sorts of other stressful incidents, for example unmanageable workloads, unfamiliar colleagues and new working hours.

Perhaps change has got a bad reputation, though. Is it possible to welcome change as if we were still five? We might not be able to recreate that feeling of wonder, but what if we could face change with the attitude of: 'wow something new that's fun,' it would feel good, right?

Given change is always going to happen, developing the most positive attitude possible gives you the best chance of maintaining your own happiness.

We will all be faced at some time with changes which are going to happen however much we like or dislike them. At some point we are all likely to face: job change, promotion, a career break or sideways step, and retirement. Some you will be dreading others you may welcome. You may even feel differently about them at different stages of your life. But you will handle this change better, make the best choices for you at the time and get the most out of both the transition and the new situation if you feel in as much control as possible. This means that even if your choices are limited (and they are never infinite) you have made the best choices you can.

Try this mind exercise which may lead you in directions you haven't thought about. The important thing here is to let your imagination run wild, so don't worry if you are creating a world which you know doesn't exist in reality.

Help yourself: the path

Imagine you are walking up a steep hill. The path becomes narrower and more difficult, it is rocky and you have to watch where you put your feet. A mist comes down then you can only see a few feet in front of you.

Then the path levels out and you find yourself walking on a wider easier path, the mist clears and you look up to a bright blue sky.

You realise you are at the top of a hill. The mist is behind you and ahead you can see clearly. You notice a comfortable seat and sit down and relax and enjoy the sun. You look at the ground beneath you and notice different plants and grasses, so many colours, so many textures. Then you raise your eyes and look around you. From your high vantage point you can see a long way. And you notice something else. From where you are there are many paths down the hill. Some are wide, others are narrow, some are straight, others meander, some even disappear into a thicket or wood. And they have different destinations. With some you can see where they go, with others they are too long.

Take some time to explore these paths. Set off along one which seems attractive and see what you find. If you want,then come back to the starting point on the hill and explore another.

Keep going. Who knows what you will find.

Just let yourself drift and daydream and enjoy the experience. When you feel you have done enough take a deep breath and stretch. Perhaps stand up and walk around for a while. (The purpose of this is to change your mental state and get you back into rational thinking mode.) Then reflect on what you found on your paths.

- *You are looking for general patterns here, to inform you of what feels right for you when you make choices about a change. So you might ask yourself questions such as*
  - *Is it busy or quiet?*
  - *Are there people around or is it just me?*
  - *Is it familiar or very new?*
  - *Are there many paths or one clear path?*
  - *Am I led to scenarios about my work or about other things?*
  - *Do things feel structured or free-flowing?*

(This is just a list to get you started, ask what feels important for you and you will begin to build up a strong sense about what you don't mind changing and what you really hate. In many circumstances you may not be able to stop change, but you may be able to make choices which steer towards those things you don't mind too much rather than things you hate.
So what you find can inform your choices, it can also give

you information about how you will react to some of those big life changes which will come your way.)

***

Go with what suits you
Let's take one example, that of taking a career break because you are starting a family. If you love being in a team and value structure and implementing a plan, for example then you may find your coming career break a daunting prospect.

You may fear the isolation and the unpredictability and lack of routine which goes with a new baby. Accept that this is you and look to how you can ameliorate that change.

Perhaps you will need the mother and baby group more than most and you will already be reading all the books in detail and have your questions for the health visitor ready.

That is you, so go with it, enjoy becoming an expert and making a plan. Look out for as much outside interaction as you can get. Then the change will feel more comfortable and you can enjoy the good bit, that lovely new baby.

Case study Mary

Mary has been working full time for the last 20 years, since her children went to secondary school. She is now 58 and came to see me because she was sleeping badly for the first time in her life. She told me she was feeling increasingly anxious and it was getting worse by the day. This was making her frustrated and annoyed with herself. She said: "I have been careful with money and saved so I could have a good retirement and I should be looking forward to it, but I am getting more and more worried. I lay awake at night wondering about what I will be doing in a year's time. I want to be happy and I keep telling myself I can be, but I can't get any pictures in my head."

I used a technique called 'the miracle question', to help Mary use her feelings and acceptance of those feelings as a guide to what she wanted. I asked her to 'imagine you woke up tomorrow morning and in the night a miracle had happened and you know exactly what you want to do. How would you know something had changed, what would you be thinking and feeling, what would you be doing?' Mary said going to work, finishing at lunchtime helping with the grandchildren and singing in the choir. It was a real lightbulb moment for her. She didn't want to stop work she just wanted to work less! Once she grasped this her anxiety receded.

She said she felt a bit foolish in that she hadn't come to this obvious answer herself. I wasn't surprised though. It's very easy to get fixated on what other people say you should want or what society seems to expect. This process can be slow and insidious and often it is unconscious. By following what seems to be the established pattern or what others expect of you, the result is a wrong fit for you. Often the first you know about it is when you begin to feel anxious and unhappy.

At that point stop and make the change work for you.

This is what Mary did. She talked to her family, and to her surprise found everyone very supportive of her desire to keep working. She had built up a barrier which wasn't really there.

A year later Mary is working part time as a job share in a different organisation. She is happy and contented, much less tired and doesn't feel anxious. "I'm not sure how long I will do this but that's okay. I am happy to take every day as it comes," she says.

Case study Ben

Ben has been taking time to look after his two children. He and his partner Bob adopted a three-year-old boy two years ago and are now in the process of adopting a little girl of four. Bob runs his own IT company and took time out when their son arrived, but in a tougher environment both feel that Bob cannot afford to do this again. Ben has decided to take a career break from his role as an emergency nurse.

He says:"I plan to be away for a least a couple of years, until both children are in school full time. Bob and I have discussed the possibility of me going back to work at weekends. This would mean I had more time in the week to be with the kids but obviously it would cut into family weekend time.

"I have loved the buzz of emergency nursing but I wonder if it is the best thing for me with young children. I don't relish coming home from a Saturday night shift and falling into bed while the rest of the family is off to the seaside. Having more time in the week sounds good but then I think, once the kids are in school I will just be rattling around the house on my own. I have thought of moving into another specialty but I think this move would need to be permanent and that frightens me. It might sound ageist but I cannot see myself dealing with the Saturday night rush at 50 or 55."

Ben said he was feeling 'a bit anxious' but wanted help to sort out what to do, 'a bit of life coaching,' as he put it. He said the changes going on were very welcome but, "It's made me think very deeply about who I am and what I want."

I used the path technique with Ben and he explored many scenarios and events and came to a firm conclusion. He said: "I know even more clearly what I most want to be - a good parent. a good partner and a good nurse. I naturally put them in that order somehow and I know that is the right order, at least for a while."

Ben and I spent another session together where we used visualisation in hypnosis to explore his core values at work, as that was the area where change was feeling the most uncomfortable for him.

We found what he liked most was a feeling of tasks completed, he found this worked for him as an emergency nurse as he felt he could complete a patient intervention and then move on to the next patient.

That sense of completion plus the buzz and liveliness of his environment were what he really enjoyed. He began to see that theatre nursing might be a good sideways move which would fit with his values and give him a work schedule which would better fit with family life.

***

Chapter Six

New jobs, different roles, finding what suits you

Changing circumstances, stretching your knowledge, working overseas, a new challenge; these are just some of the reasons you might want to change your job. Here are some ways you can make sure you make the right choice.

In a previous chapter we have talked about burnout and hopefully you can now recognise the danger signs and do something about it. Yet there are times when you might feel that you want to make a change in your career, even when everything is going well in your current role. It's not surprising that we all hanker after changes from time to time, given that we change throughout our lives.

How much do you change?
It may sound obvious to point out that we are always changing, but in fact change is so difficult for us to accept that it has a psychological label all to itself. It is named the 'end of history illusion'. What this says is that we all, at whatever stages of our lives, believe we have reached our optimum level and won't change much more.

So why do we do this, can it be true? Three researchers,

Jordi Quoidbach, Daniel Gilbert and Timothy Wilson have looked at these questions in detail and investigated how people perceive themselves changing.

They asked more than 19,000 people if they had changed much in the last decade and if they expected to change much in the decade to come. They asked these people about their personality traits, their favourite foods, holiday destinations and hobbies. Then they published their findings in the journal *Science* in 2013.

They found that wherever people were in their lives at present, whether young, middle-aged or old, most believed that they had changed a lot up to this point, but now things were pretty fixed and they would remain essentially the same person for the rest of their life.

Daniel Gilbert summed up the findings: "Middle aged people . . . often look back on our teenage selves with some mixture of amusement and chagrin. What we never seem to realise is that our future selves will look back and think the very same thing about us. At every age we think we're having the last laugh and at every age we are wrong."

The three researchers speculated about why this is so, and suggested that it might be because we get a deep sense of satisfaction from thinking we are at our very best now, and so we foster the illusion. Another idea they came up with was that we find it easy to remember what has happened to us, so can quite accurately recall the changes we have made, but we find it much harder to imagine the future and what changes are coming up. This means we find it hard to speculate on our future choices as we carry on through life.

What changes and what stays the same
This fascinating piece of research is important when we are considering big life changes. If you are going to change as much in the next ten years as in the past ten, how do you

know what will be best for you, what will make you most happy? Or if you are perfectly happy in your job now how do you know that this will continue if you are going to change so much?Eeek! That sounds like making any rational change is impossible doesn't it?

There is a natural guide, however, and that is about knowing your basic personality type and how that fits the framework of your career.

Because nursing is such a demanding job, both emotionally and physically, this 'do I really want to be doing this?' feeling probably comes up more frequently than in other careers. Change happens, so it helps if you can embrace it and use it as a positive drive and development. Adapting your career can build on the skills and learning that you already have. So think about how you might use all those caring skills and expert knowledge in a different environment.

Think back to what we learned in the first chapter of this book, where we looked at what makes a fulfilling life. Many of these things apply to all of us, they are part of being human. But we can work on and refine these big things to craft them to our personality and the realistic expectations we can have for our own lives. We should each be aiming for a role which fits our basic personality, but allows space to grow and develop, and we might not know how that growth and development is going to be.

So is there a way of telling the difference between a transitory feeling which might suggest you need a holiday, and your mind and your body telling you it is time for a serious change of direction?

What average looks like
Let's start with the average. This sounds strange doesn't it? After all who wants to be average? No-one, which is probably why study after study has found we are all big-heads,

constantly over-rating our positive qualities while insisting that we score below average on negative qualities.

But remember we learned in chapter one that an important habit of happy fulfilled people is honesty? So be honest about your capabilities. You are much more likely be to quite good at what you do than the very best in the whole world. So start looking at how most people, good but not spectacularly good, perform a role you think you would like to do. Is this like you? Are the people who are happy doing this like you? Would you get on with them if you saw them every day? What does their typical day look like and does that suit your life, the types of commitments you have, your biorhythms and your life preferences?

Now, do a thought experiment. Ask, "If I had a really bad day how much would I then hate the job, would I be prepared to stick at it?" If you would, then you are moving in a good direction for you. Once you have done this you can clarify things more by focusing your attention on the different areas of your life in turn. This can throw light on whether your motivation to change is driven by your job, other areas of your life, or how the two interact (including your preferred work/life balance).

Sorting out your feelings
So let's start by thinking about your job. Take some quiet time and consider the things on the list below. Don't treat this as box ticking, there are no right and wrong answers, it is a way of finding out what matters most to you.

Do the exercise when you are feeling reasonably relaxed and reflective – this is not the time for quick unconsidered decisions. So as you read down the list, notice how you are feeling – you are likely to find that some things make you inwardly (or even outwardly) shout 'Yes that's right!'

Other things on the list might not appear very important

or relevant for you. Jot down your feelings and immediate thoughts – how you feel, what are your strongest feelings, what really matters.

Don't worry at this stage about what is practical or possible. It is much better to get the clearest idea about how you feel and what you would like to do and *then* look at what that means in practical terms.

Also consider whether you want just to look at your next move or whether you want to plan further down the line, into the next decade of your life and career or even further. Again, there is no right or wrong about this – if you are young and absolutely convinced that several children are going to be part of your life in the future then you might want to plan ahead. If you are the sort of person who takes the view that you don't know what life holds, you may want to look just at the next step.

Consider your life, your job, your personal life and how the two interact. How are they looking to you at the moment? Go through the list below and you will get a clearer idea.

Challenges and development
● Do you feel you are given the support, training and help you need to keep up with new developments in your particular area?
● Have you been given a chance to build up expertise in your area and is this recognised in your organisation?
● Have you made an impact where you work, are things different because you are there?

Prospects for advancement
● Is there a realistic chance of you getting a promotion in a time frame which is suitable for you? (If that is important for you – not everyone wants promotion and there is nothing

wrong with that).

Money matters
- Can you live as you want on your salary now and in the future?

Your work environment
- Do you like and value your colleagues and do they like and value you?
- Do you respect your managers and think they are doing a good job?
- Are your values reflected in the values of your workplace?
- Is the pace of work suitable for your personality?

Your environment
- Are you happy with the key relationships in your life?
- Are you happy in the town, city or village where you live?
- Are you happy in the street or immediate community where you live?
- Are you happy in your house or flat?
- Do you have friends or family with whom you share your feelings?

Your work and life
- Does your job allow enough time for you to see your family and friends?
- Will this be true in the future? (if you decide to have children, or when your children leave home for example.)
- Is there something you would really like to do outside work (a sporting challenge, an artistic venture, or volunteering for example) and does your work allow space for this?
- Does your work allow you to use what you regard as your greatest strengths as a person?

Where to focus

After you have reflected on these questions, you should have a clearer idea about whether it is your job, the rest of your life, or how the two are interacting which is the most important thing to change.

Of course this is never completely clear-cut, but nearly always you will find that one of these areas stands out from the others. This is where you should start to make changes.

If it is your work, or the interaction between your work and the rest of your life, then it might be time to think of a career shift. So read on. . .

Changing the course of your career is obviously a big decision so you want to make sure that you are getting it right.

What's the problem?

Let's start by clarifying what is wrong. If you are feeling it is time for a change in your career then begin by focusing on what is unsatisfying in your work life at present. Sometimes it can be one thing that is frustrating you and affecting how you feel about a role which you actually like. If this thing is temporary or you can change it then that may be a better option than moving job or even changing your whole career trajectory.

Clarifying your thoughts about your work

Are there some parts of your current role that you particularly like or dislike? Has that changed recently and if so do you know why?

If you know something you really dislike about your role then ask yourself: 'Could I (in principle) do my job without this part that I dislike?'

If you could, then ask yourself the following questions:

1) If your job was without the element you dislike how would it be different? Think about this in detail and imagine what

an average day would be like. How does that day differ from your average day now?

2) How would *you* be without the thing you dislike? How are you looking, feeling and behaving? What are you doing which you cannot do at the moment?

You will get one of two outcomes from this exercise.

A) The 'all is basically good' outcome

All is good. By thinking about your work without the dislikeable thing you find you feel happy, full of energy, optimistic. You then need to ask how you can replicate this in reality. Can you discuss with your manager, or your team about making changes which would minimise the dislikeable thing, or make it less intrusive?

Or it might be that you can make this future happen by changing department or moving team. Or perhaps you can investigate opportunities to do the same job in a different workplace. You will know and feel more confident to plan your future now you know what needs to change and what you want to stay the same.

A word of warning here. When we have a vague feeling that something is not right about our place of work it is very easy to focus on something which is in our face, part of our everyday experience rather than looking for underlying causes. Living a busy life every day it is easy to get caught up in the minutiae of life.

If you are feeling frustrated at work, a natural tendency is to focus on the little everyday things. So perhaps a lot of your energy has been taken up by how annoying Dave the Doctor is. You know him, he waltzes onto the ward as if he's God's gift and you immediately feel the stress response kicking in. Your main dislikeable thing has become Dave and most of your feelings of frustration and even anger are directed towards him.

This might be the whole truth for you, but it is probably not. It is more likely that Dave is a symptom of something else (lack of control on your ward, feeling you are not recognised for your skills, would be examples) rather than the main cause of your uncomfortable feelings. It is worth looking deeper. If you are feeling this then you may be moving towards the need for a bigger change.

So be honest, if Dave the Doctor was removed (in whichever manner you find most satisfying! - I don't need to know more) would things be hunky dory? Chances are you will say - well probably not. If this resonates with you, it is worth at least looking at some bigger changes.

B) The 'needing a bigger change' outcome

This is when you realise it isn't just that dislikeable thing, but wider issues which are bothering you and making you frustrated in your current career. In this case it is perhaps time you looked around to develop your nursing role in other directions. This result might have surprised you. Remember though, deciding to change jobs does not have to come from negative feelings. There is usually some level of frustration or a feeling that something is not quite right, but there can also be a reaching out, a yearning for something different, challenging and fresh.

Push and pull factors

You may find yourself experiencing conflicting emotions. Some will be negative, you want to get away from your current situation, and some will be positive; you will want to go towards a better situation. These emotions are reflecting real things in your world.

There will be 'push factors': things you don't like are pushing you away from your current role and into something new, and 'pull factors' – positive gains pulling you towards a change even if you are not sure what you want that change to be yet.

Making any career change is usually a mixture of the positive and negative emotions and the push and pull factors. This can feel confusing and conflicted, but there are ways of untangling the emotional spaghetti. It can help to write at this stage. Writing is a very good way of sorting out feelings and seeing something on paper can give it solidity, a reality which it may have lacked up until now.

Untangling your emotions
Make a list in two columns – what you want to leave behind in your work and what you want to take with you into a new role. Your list will be yours, unique and individual but it might help you to get started by reading the next section on pull and push factors.

Frequent push factors include:
- Boredom in your current role
- Lack of training opportunities
- Lack of promotion chances
- Feeling bullied or put upon
- Tension with colleagues

Frequent pull factors include:
- Wanting to try a different healthcare environment
- Wanting more flexibility and more control over hours
- Wanting to travel or move to a different city
- Wanting more responsibility and control over the environment you work in
- Wanting to work with a completely different patient group
- Wanting to work with people who are not sick
- Wanting to work outside of a healthcare environment

Pull factors frequently become stronger as your life-experience changes. So, for example, having a family may pull you towards roles which offer fewer or more family-friendly hours. Or you may be getting older and thinking about retirement, but still feel you have a lot to give to the profession. In this case perhaps you may be pulled towards contract or consultancy work.

Another big pull factor can be growing confidence as you become more experienced in the profession. You may feel you are ready to take on new challenges or that you have exhausted the possibilities in one area.

As most decisions include both pull and push factors it is worth considering the balance for you. Pull feels good – optimistic looking to the future, making good changes. Push can feel more difficult – like running away from something, or feeling trapped and unhappy in your current situation and giving in by deciding to leave.

This tension between push and pull can sometimes feel very uncomfortable and may even appear to be getting in the way of making a decision.

Value fear
It's about resolution and integration and acknowledging your negative feelings as well as the positive. Forget the slogans such as 'feel the fear and do it anyway' – this is your life we are talking about here, not a bungee jump. The fear will be reflecting something important for you and you can integrate the positive aspects of this into your feelings and then into your plans.

Value fear, it is a vital part of our psychological make-up and an important factor in making any major decision. Often this is related to your security and emotional and physical comfort. As a species we are pretty hard-wired to avoid change, for most of our human existence it was best to stick with the band, not to wander away from the village as to do so risked starvation or being eaten by wild animals.

On the other hand none of us would be here unless our ancestors had been a pretty adventurous bunch, which they obviously were; they spread out all over the globe after all, literally walking into the unknown.

So there is a conflict there, range far and wide or stay close to home. Just reading that phrase may have elicited some strong feelings in you. Are you excited by 'range far and wide' or comforted by 'stay close at home'? Save that feeling and respect it, do not try to make yourself something you are not.

You will know if you are naturally a person who values familiarity, close and well-established relationships and a known work environment. On the other hand, you might be a person who is easily bored, who looks out new relationships and who is never happier than during the first days of a new job or a new project. As far as possible go with your natural preferences.

It can be more complicated than that, though. Sometimes you will want to change, or have to change even though it is scary. Sometimes your fear can be a manifestation of low self esteem or a belief that you won't succeed, and that is not very useful. What we need to do then is to respect the fear and work to integrate it, taking the useful parts and discarding the parts which are holding you back.

Help Yourself: focus on what you think you want and see what happens

Try this technique to help free up your unconscious and integrate your push and pull factors. You can then end up with a realistic plan for your future which fits with you and takes account of your fears and concerns. What do you want? Sum this up in one phrase. Do you think you can make this happen? Rate this on a scale of 1 to 10 (with 1 being low and 10 high). Now let that fade and imagine as strongly as you can where you would like to be in your career in one year's time. Make this imagining as strong as you can and use all your senses, so make a bright picture and add some sound, a background melody perhaps or people's voices, even your own. Let your body feel how you feel, are you excited, anticipatory, calm, happy? Don't try too hard, just let the feelings grow.

Now focus on your hands while keeping that imagining going as strongly as you can. Start with your hands on your knees and then let your hands move in any way they want to reflect how you want to be. You might find your hands spread out wide or they might move up and down at different speeds or clasp together. Often they will feel as if they are acting independently of you – don't worry just let your hands go wherever feels right. Once you feel comfortable begin to experiment. Consciously move your hands while focusing on that future you want, you may want to make patterns in the air or form your hands into a shape. Keep doing this until you feel that your hand movements are representing what this future could be. Now move your attention and think about what is holding you back. This could be fear of change, feeling comfortable where you are, worrying about what others will think. Whatever it is focus your hands and let them move in a way which represents that limitation. Again just let your hands make shapes, move as they want, go wherever feels right. When you feel that your hand movements or shapes are representing those factors then consciously move your hands until you feel they are really representing how you

147

are holding yourself back. (Perhaps they are clasped tight or palms facing down or clamped hard on your knees).

Now make the first movement again (the 'what you want' one) and then switch to the second movement. Make each movement switching from one to the other several times (between 10 and 20). Notice that the 'holding back' position begins to become weaker while the ' what you want' position begins to change slightly. As you do this let your mind clear, don't try to concentrate or problem-solve, just let your mind flit around and settle where it wants. You may notice your imagining of the future changes to deal with or even incorporate those things that might be holding you back.

Relax and imagine that future again as clearly as you can. You may find you have solved what was holding you back. Focus on what you want. And ask yourself the question again. Do you think you can make this happen? Rate this on a scale of 1 to 10 (with 1 being low and 10 high)?

It will get higher as you clarify your own thoughts and feelings and focus on your strengths.

***

**** Case study Julie ****

I used this technique with a client (Julie). Julie is a 40-year-old nurse based in a teaching hospital. She had worked in a variety of hospital settings and was currently working on a busy general ward (where she had spent several years). She came to see me because she was feeling anxious, tired and was beginning to find work 'too much, it's too hard' she would say. When we talked further she said she felt her 'sparkle' had gone and this was affecting how she related to her patients and her colleagues.

She felt ashamed that she was often snappy with her colleagues. She was clear that she didn't hate her job, she just didn't feel that interest and enthusiasm which she remembered fondly from her past. Her working conditions were broadly similar, although she had recently gone through a restructuring process and moved wards. Her family situation was changing as her youngest child started secondary school and her eldest prepared to leave home to go to university.

Julie found it quite difficult to acknowledge her feelings. She kept saying: "I am lucky, I have a good job and a nice family, perhaps I expect too much." We decided to use the technique I described above to explore what was going on.

Julie had a vague image of where she wanted her career to be, it was somewhere quieter, in a country environment. She could hear her footsteps as she walked along quiet carpeted corridors. She met colleagues as she walked and everyone spoke in a gentle considered tone. She felt very comfortable and quietly happy in this situation. When she focused on her hands she found herself putting one on top of the other and clasping them gently. She said this felt very warm and comforting – 'gentle' was the word she used. She moved her hands about a little, wiggling her fingers, and then settled back in the original position, one on top of the other gently clasping, because that felt right for her.

She then focused on what was holding her back; she clenched her fists tightly and bumped them together. She moved between the two movements for about five minutes. Slowly her fists relaxed until she found her hands settling with one hand on top of the other with the top hand slightly clasped. I asked how she felt about this, "I want something gentle, but I need a bit of effort to get there," she replied.

When she imagined the future scene again it was sharper and clearer. She felt she was in a private hospital in an outpatients or a short-stay department or setting, perhaps where minor surgical procedures were being performed. She was walking along a corridor to visit a patient who was about to be discharged and she wanted to ensure that he was happy and comfortable and ready to leave. She was thinking about helping this patient and then what she was doing for the rest of the day.

She was looking forward to a meeting to discuss a new procedure which the hospital was shortly to carry out and on which she would be the nurse lead. "I won't be bored'" she said. She recognised that being bored after working in a busy NHS hospital had been a fear. Now she saw that if she chose well it did not have to be that way.

Shortly after this session she applied for a 4-day-a-week position at a local private hospital. She got it and describes herself as being fulfilled and happy in her job.

***

Stories from a nursing life: Paul Jebb

"Understanding how people connect helps you care"

In a career which has taken him from the wards to a secondment with NHS England, Paul Jebb found learning from strong role models enabled him to mentor and inspire others.

When did you decide to become a nurse?
My dad was involved in a road traffic accident in 1988. That was my first introduction to seeing how nurses worked as part of a team. I witnessed the whole course of my dad's recovery, treatment, rehabilitation and home care, and through that I realised the depth and breadth of what nurses do. It sparked my interest in health care.

What was the appeal?
Seeing how nurses dealt with patients and their families really impacted on me, plus the variety of challenges they had to deal with daily. For example, when my dad came home from hospital, it wasn't possible to get him and his wheelchair into the house. But the district nurse who was there to meet him came up with a plan to go through next

door's garden and into our house via the back door. It worked.

Did you consider any other careers? If so, what were they and why did you reject them?

I did look at medicine, but at the age of 16, having left school, the last thing I wanted to do was A levels, so I topped up my GCSEs and then reviewed what my options were.

How did you decide which branch of nursing to go into?

I did consider children's nursing, but decided that I may have more long term career options if I did adult nursing.

What were the highs and lows of being a nursing student when you trained?

Lots of highs - election to RCN Council as Chair of RCN Students, being involved as a student in shaping nursing's future, connecting with others across the international nursing community. The best bits were caring for people and I can still remember some of them, their names and the surgery they went through. These people kept me going through the tough times. I did fail a couple of exams and had to resit, this was hard as it added to the pressure of the course and the pressure of part time work to supplement my bursary.

Where was your first job after qualifying?

I was a staff nurse on a general/ear, nose and throat (ENT) surgical ward at Blackpool Victoria Hospital.

How did it compare with your expectations?

I didn't feel at all prepared for the business of acute care, and the variety of expectations from patients and staff as well as the demands on me.

How did your career develop post qualification?
I became a charge nurse at Blackpool and then moved to another ward where I became a manager (surgical directorate) in July 2000. From there, I was seconded for a year to become Recruitment and Retention Facilitator in the Directorate of Governance, followed by a variety of senior management positions in which I was able to lead on a variety of important projects, including implementation of the Productive Ward scheme across the trust. An important move for me was the promotion to Assistant Director of Nursing/Patient Experience in 2010. I am currently seconded to NHS England. This role includes developing toolkits for commissioners to enhance experience of care, leading on 'working with people to provide a positive experience of care' action area of the National Compassion in Practice strategy, working with Institute of Healthcare Improvement to develop 'Always events', working with health care regulators to enhance experience of care strategies as well as raising the profile of experiences of care across the NHS.

Who have been the most important role models during your career? What qualities did you most admire in them?
Without naming them, I think I have been fortunate to have discovered different role models in a number of fields: politics, management, clinical practice, education. Faced with a decision to make I will often ask myself how they would have responded.

Did you ever feel that the demands of the job put you under unacceptably high levels of stress?
The role of a nurse can indeed be very stressful, not always, but it can also be very rewarding. I have always

worked with great supportive teams and had managers that looked after their staff, having a partner who is a nurse also helps as they understand the job and the need for relaxation time.

How do you deal with stress?
Making sure you have time for yourself is key; some roles have had higher stress than others. I find exercise and cycling really does clear my head and helps me stay in control. Cycling out in the country, with no one around is very relaxing. Even being on my bike or at the gym is enough, but it is important to take that time.

What strategies did you use to get you through the most challenging times in your career?
It is paramount that you are honest with yourself and if things are getting too much to address these.

What are you most proud of in terms of your career as a nurse?
I think I am proud of how I have inspired others. I find mentoring and coaching really rewarding and learning is key to developing ourselves and the care we deliver.

How has being a nurse affected other areas of your life such as family and friendships?
Juggling work and life isn't easy, especially since children have come along, bringing taxi duties. No matter what role I have had I have made time for friends and family. Some friendships have fizzled due to work demands on both sides, but keeping contact even if it just a call at Christmas is essential.

What would you say are the main qualities needed to be a good nurse?
Being human and understanding how humans connect, and communicate, is paramount. That enables you to build a relationship so that you can develop the caring role with the people you are looking after as well as their families and other staff members.

In your opinion, how has nursing changed since you were starting out?
I think nursing will always be nursing, the profession has developed and has had more demands put on it, but fundamental nursing care has remained and is respected.

Would you recommend nursing to anyone considering a career in the profession today?
Absolutely! I can honestly say I have enjoyed my career through the tough times and the happy times.

Key Facts

When did you train as a nurse?
Started a diploma programme in 1993 qualified in 1996

Where?
University of Central Lancashire

Qualifications
MA, BSc (Hons), DipHE

Current role
Experience of Care Professional lead, NHS England

Chapter Seven

How to become the master of your workplace culture

Can you develop a mindset which will enable you to get the very best from your colleagues? In most cases the answer is 'yes if you know how.' And it will make you happier and more effective.

One of the best things about nursing is the opportunities it offers to move around, to change jobs and to learn about new areas. For many of you, this variety may have been one of the main reasons you were attracted to nursing in the first place. A lot of the time this will be a wholly positive part of your career. But there can be times when a new environment, or changes in an existing environment, leave you feeling like a fish out of water.

In this chapter I want to help you swim happily, whatever the workplace culture you find yourself in, and learn how to shape it and change it when you spot something wrong.

The more you understand and the more adept you are at making the work experience as fulfilling and supportive as it can be, the happier you will be at work.

Also, if you recognise what a healthy workplace culture looks like you will be better at spotting when it is not there. Poor workplace cultures can be at best depressing places and, at worst, fertile ground for bullying.

Building a healthy workplace culture
Nurses are great people watchers; empathy and fascination with people are also factors that may have brought you to the profession. You probably use your people-watching skills everyday to build up the best relationships you can with your patients or clients. So why not broaden these skills and use them to develop strong relationships and networks which will make you happier at work and help develop your career?

Be aware that you need the right resources to be happy at work and it is usually other people who control those resources. Know what you need and who has the power to provide you with access to it. Then notice that sometimes people are acting as individuals and sometimes as part of a group or network. If you need to join or relate to one or more of these networks then find out how you are going to do it, and who are the key people to smooth your path.

This approach may sound rather cold and instrumental, but remember that if you do this well, you will feel happier and more relaxed, you will be a nicer person to be around for your workmates and you will deliver a better service for your patients. Start by developing a healthy mindset for yourself. That is yours, in your control and no-one can take it away from you. Take a little time every day to remind yourself of your goals and enjoy the people around you. You will begin to learn a lot about them. Then ask yourself:

• Who has real influence, who has paper authority but not real influence, who is able to influence the overall culture (this is not always the person with the formal power)?
• Who is speaking to whom? What groups are there? Which do you want to be part of, are there any you want to avoid?
• What do you have to offer? Who is the most important

person in your network? Can you work with them so you give your optimum performance? What needs to happen to bring this about?

- Do you have all the resources you need to do your job well? Do you have access to the information you need? If not who does, do you know them?
- Are there people who are stopping you achieving what you need to do? What are their goals, can their goals be aligned with yours?

Everyone is interesting

Try to develop the most open and embracing attitude you can. A good way of starting this is to regard everyone as interesting. That's it, interesting: whether or not they are good at their job, whether or not you get on with them, they will have things about them which are interesting.

If someone is annoying you, when they are doing that thing you really hate, or that you find a complete mystery, imagine that you are leaning back, stroking your chin like the wise old owl you are (on the inside at least) and saying to yourself: "mmm . . . that's an interesting way of doing that. I would never have seen things that way." Think of humanity as an endless game of different ways of going about things. Soon you will be adept at spotting the different styles people use to do their work.

Different people, different styles

There is a whole industry in management psychology about spotting different personality types and how they affect people's relationships with each other in the workplace.

Most of these models are a bit too rigid and often don't take enough account of how people will shift and change as their environment changes. However, if you've never considered your workplace in this light they can be a great way of getting you started in this 'aren't we all different' mindset. One of the best known is that devised by Meredith Belbin. He identified nine team roles which were needed for effective performance and noted that certain individuals are more suited to some than others. He also noted that each role has a downside, what he calls allowable weaknesses. Here are the basic types, and their weaknesses:

- Shaper: Challenges the team to improve, but can be aggressive if things stall.
- Implementer: Puts ideas into action, but can resist change.
- Completer/Finisher: Ensures tasks are completed well, but can display perfectionism.
- Co-ordinator: Acts as a chairperson, but can over-delegate their own responsibilities.
- Team Worker: Encourages co-operation, but can be indecisive when tough decisions are needed.
- Resource Investigator: Looks for new ways of finding resources, but can be forgetful about following-up.
- Plant: Presents new ideas and approaches, but can be too unorthodox and forgetful.
- Monitor/Evaluator: Analyses the options, but can be slow and critical.
- Specialist: Provides specialised skills, but often doesn't notice the bigger picture.

You can probably see people you work with here. Can you see yourself? Can you feel where you fit in and where other people fit as well? If you feel a strong connection to one of these types, then you can probably understand why a colleague who fits the profile for another type might get up your nose sometimes. Can you now see how useful they are to the team?

Celebrate difference

With this sort of knowledge, you can begin to value difference. You probably do this better than most people anyway, as it is part of your skills as a nurse. However, none of us are saints, and it seems to be a pretty universal trait that we get on best with those who are most like us. This basic trait is often exacerbated when we are busy, need to get the job done and don't have time to reflect on the wonderful possibilities of difference.

Tools like the Belbin system above can help us to get some understanding of how differences benefit us all. If you put that difference, and its benefits, at the centre of your new mindset then you can say much more easily: 'we see things differently' or 'I know my way annoys you, but let's agree to differ'. Perhaps you can talk about how different strengths benefit the whole team, the work environment and patient care. Don't be afraid to be specific.

For example, if you are a 'Resource Investigator' there is no harm in saying to your 'Shaper' colleague: "You may be very goal-orientated and focused on us developing that new strategy, and I understand how important that is, even though I couldn't do it myself. I am different, concerned about where we can find the resources to put that strategy in place, so how do we work together on this?" Done well, with openness and respect, you can get to a very powerful vision and take even more powerful action together.

Be flexible

Ask yourself, 'Will the world end if someone does things differently?' Sometimes, you will have to stand your ground, where patient safety is concerned for example, but often, however much someone else's way annoys you it is better to let it go, and even take an inquiring look to see if that way works.

Be a constant coach. Take the attitude that you are always learning and so is everyone else in your team. Take every opportunity to say: "That's interesting, I never thought of doing that." Perhaps set yourself a target of saying this several times a week, then you will have to look for those times when people are doing things differently, you might be surprised at how that changes your outlook. When you spot these new ways of doing things, ask questions and take the chance to praise others, say: "What is it you do that means bad-tempered patient x is all smiles when you come along?"

Perhaps this all sounds a bit sugar candy to you, as if it would only work in a perfect world. If you are feeling like this, it might be that your workplace or team is very difficult in which case some of the techniques below might help. It may be that your workplace is so dysfunctional and aggressive that you will be shot down for doing this, in which case you need to take more action, including taking the matter up formally and even changing jobs. No-one deserves or needs to work in an aggressive environment where you cannot grow and learn.

Bullying environments and how to cope

Bullying does not exist in a vacuum, sometimes all it takes is for good people to do nothing.

We all have a picture in our heads of what bullying is: perhaps being shouted at and having our work achievements constantly undermined. This certainly is bullying, but it is not the only form. There are other less obvious behaviours which cause just as much damage and should also be identified as bullying. Behaviours such as withholding information that you need to do you job well or excluding you from decision making are just as undermining and as likely to cause you psychological harm, and they are harder to recognise.

I am going to concentrate on what you can do to protect yourself psychologically and emotionally if you are being bullied. You may need to do more than this. If you are being bullied, it might be necessary to go to your union, staff association or manager and report the problem formally. If the situation doesn't resolve itself, and you feel there is no realistic chance of improving things, you may need to consider changing your job.

The long-term effects of bullying can take a terrible toll on your mental and physical health and no job is worth that. One of the worst aspects of being bullied is that it robs you of your confidence and motivation. It also forces you to alter your behaviour so in the end you are behaving in ways which you don't like, didn't choose and are not doing you any good. Often, in an attempt to protect yourself you will end up hiding from the bully or bullies.

You may believe that the only way you can cope is to keep your head down and keep out of the way and this will almost certainly make you miserable and may end up damaging your career. It can also make the problem worse as the bully will usually perceive your weakness and increase the attack.

Bullying can happen anywhere, but it is particularly present wherever people are oppressed, as is often the case for nurses. "The female-dominated profession of nursing has typically fallen under male-dominated groups of physicians and administrators in the power structure of health care systems," says Amy Glenn Vega, author of *Lions and Tigers and Nurses*. "Theoretically, members of an oppressed group will turn on each other and use violence as a way to achieve power over their peers."

The reasons for this are complex but many researchers have found that gender and medical dominance certainly add to the problem (Duffy 1995, Hockley 2002). There is some evidence that nurses internalise this inferiority and this can lead to many problems, including depression and stress. (Freshwater 2000).

The 'power map' in most organisations in which you work as a nurse is likely to be very complex. Shifting alliances, different pressures from managerial and professional structures and inter-professional rivalries, misunderstandings and different world views all conspire against a transparent culture in which people know what their goals are and can measure their success.

Name the problem
Remember bullying is a behaviour – you can choose how you react to it. The first thing you need to do is name the problem. Just saying to yourself: 'I am being bullied and I am not prepared to put up with it,' is liberating. It's not you, the problem is out there, not in your head. It is amazing how making the decision to refuse to internalise bullying can strengthen you. It is best if you can do this in a supportive setting, perhaps opening up to family or friends about what is going on.

Then take a long and honest look at your situation and how you are behaving.

Let's be very clear here, I am not saying you are doing anything wrong or that you are responsible for the bullying, but bullying can be so demoralising and confidence-wrecking that it is very easy to begin to behave in ways which are sending out loud messages that you have low self esteem and will not stand up for yourself. And this of course can make the bullying even worse. It will also make you feel rotten.

If you have been trying to keep your head down as a way of coping with the bullying, you may be internalising the message that you are doing something wrong. You are not, the bully is. However, you may be sending out the subconscious message that it is your fault. Your self-esteem may have fallen and you can lose confidence in your abilities. It might help to look at it this way. Everything you do is sending out some message. You cannot exist in the world and not communicate. You have no choice over that, but you do have a choice about what messages you send out.

Being strong and confident is sending messages, and so is hiding and keeping your head down. Each is sending a whole range of verbal and non-verbal signals about what you think about yourself. Every time you speak to people around you, what you say will be reinforced by your body language and your general demeanour.

If you can change, so the message you are sending out is that you are a confident person who expects to be treated well and will not put up with any s**t, then you are doing something which may protect you against the bullying. And even if it doesn't, you will have done something to help yourself. Your mind, your thoughts, your body language and your behaviour constantly impact on each other.

So if you can deliberately change your behaviour to appear more confident and assertive then your thoughts will follow.

If you cannot avoid sending messages, and you cannot, then doesn't it make sense to choose what messages you send? Choose how you want to react and what you want others to think of you. Wouldn't that lead to a better outcome for you?

This doesn't always come easy and it may not always work in that it may not always change the bullying behaviour, but if you can do it then you may begin to be able to put the bully into perspective and protect yourself more.

Getting the new mindset
It may take some time to get into this new mindset, and then

decide what to do. So put yourself first. Do not be afraid to take time off work and use this time to build your self-esteem and plan your next moves. Get your physical health checked as well, as the stress of being bullied can take its toll on you. Take legal advice or go to your union if appropriate.

If you do not take time off, look after yourself in your leisure time. Try this way of building your confidence and self esteem.

Help yourself: positive thoughts

Take yourself to a quiet place and practise relaxing breathing. First of all, take deep breaths and on the in breath push your tummy out. Then begin counting your breaths, breathing in for seven and out for eleven (or whatever feels comfortable, what is important is that the out breath is longer than the in breath). As you breathe out imagine that all the tension, every worry is leaving your body.

Say to yourself, "more relaxed" as you breathe out. Do this for a few minutes until you are feeling more relaxed. Then, starting with your feet, tense and relax all your major muscle groups.

Then create a place in your imagination which is safe and secure and lovely; it might be a memory or somewhere that you invent for yourself, do whatever feels right for you.

Notice how good you feel and congratulate yourself on making yourself feel like this. Tell yourself that you can recreate this lovely feeling anytime you want. You are going to feel healthier and fitter in every way. You will feel more alert and experience a wonderful feeling of well-being and peace with yourself.

Then say to yourself:

- From now on I focus outward.

- I focus on the positive in my life. (Imagine the most positive thing for you at the moment).
- I am optimistic and look forward to good things. (Imagine the best thing coming up for you in the next weeks).
- I am interested in the world around me and in the people around me. I am so interested in the outside world I no longer think about myself so much. (Imagine yourself interacting with others and achieving what you want).
- My mind is becoming clearer.
- I know my goals.
- My nerves are becoming steadier.
- I know I can do what I want to do.

Focus on your breathing again. As you breathe in feel that you are breathing in energy to motivate you and give you everything you want. As you do this say "I can".

This exercise should clear your mind, give you energy and help you focus on what is important to you. With that mindset and your self-esteem much recovered you can now focus outwards.

If you can, start with what you want to achieve in your job. Don't let the bully occupy centre stage in your mind. If it helps, imagine pushing them to one side leaving a nice clear space - then focus on what positive things you want to achieve in the next days and weeks. Make these realistic, and doable. When you feel you have a firm grasp on what these are, you might want to write them down.

Then ask if it is possible to communicate what you want to do to others in your team, to those with decision making power?

As you reflect, you can ask if the bully is helping or hindering this aim. The answer will usually be that they are hindering it.

But keep your focus on the aim, not the bully, if they are creeping back into the centre of your mind push them to the side again.

You now have a wider context than just the bully's behaviour. Now take a pen and begin to write

- What you want to achieve
- What you need to do this
- What needs to happen

To make this clearer, read what happened to Sarah. I especially like her story as it does not have a simple happy ending - and life is often like that isn't it?

Case study Sarah

A client of mine, Sarah, was a nurse on a day unit. She was being bullied by a co-worker. I asked her what she wanted to achieve now at work. What was a key aim for her, her patients and her team?

This is what she said:
"I want to achieve a quicker patient discharge in our unit. This fits with our overall targets and would improve patient experience. To do this I need the correct documentation. The problem is with an administrator, Hayley, who is bullying me. I need her to deliver documentation to a quicker timetable and ensure that all the information is complete and correct. This person is constantly rude to me and calls me 'Little Miss Princess, wants everything now'. She says, in a loud sing-song voice 'Princess Alert' whenever I approach her. She undermines me and talks about me in a disparaging way, making fun of my accent and appearance to colleagues. I suspect she also prioritises other teams' requirements over mine."

Sarah was very upset with the Princess comments and

was becoming very stressed and losing her confidence. On occasions, she had been reduced to tears, although she had never cried in public. After a couple of sessions, we decided to take a work-goal focused approach to this. This is what we did.

I asked Sarah to forget about Hayley for the moment and to write down in detail what she needed to do to achieve her aim. Her initial response was, I know what I need to do, and Hayley is the only thing stopping this happening.
This was interesting information indeed. I began to fire questions at Sarah. Why do you want to achieve this aim? Her answer, patient experience, it's my job, I also want to do it well so I get a chance of promotion perhaps, but at least get good feedback and respect from my managers now.

I asked: "Who else wants to achieve this aim?" Sarah thought about this for a moment, then said well everyone, the managers, the team, the patients, yes everyone. There is no downside to patients getting home more quickly and not having to hang about for ages for nothing.

Then I asked, do others in your team know where the blockage is? Sarah said they did, but everyone accepted it. It's a bit like the weather, everyone moans, but no-one thinks anything can be done about it. Did other teams or individuals have similar problems with getting necessary documentation? Sarah thought not, although she was aware that her predecessor had experienced much the same problem.

We now turned to deciding what to do.

Firstly, I asked Sarah if doing nothing was an option for her. She felt strongly that it was not, that it would go to the heart of her professional ethics to allow the situation to continue and it would harm her professional reputation and prospects in the long run.

So we decided on a plan. I began by asking Sarah to describe what she felt comfortable doing and what felt unpleasant to her. She liked devising new systems and working out better ways of doing things, in fact this was an important reason she had got the role in the first place. She disliked confrontation.

So I asked her to spend the next week producing a business case outlining why quicker discharge times were good, and a flow chart of what was needed to make this happen. As she worked on this she realised she needed information and input from other colleagues.

This presented her with a challenge and an opportunity. Should she go to these colleagues and say what she was doing? We talked about this and I encouraged her to keep a focus on the professional goal. She decided there were two key colleagues whose input was essential and she was delighted to find they were both enthusiastic about her plans, as well as giving her some new ideas. When she was happy about the plan we talked about where to go next. She felt that in 'an ideal world' she should involve Hayley, but she felt the previous hostility she had faced meant she would not cope well.

So she took her plan to her own senior manager and it went well, she was congratulated on her initiative and praised for the quality of the work. Her manager spoke, in fairly guarded terms, about 'people who don't like change' and 'blocks to doing things'. At that point Sarah took a leap: she said: 'If you mean Hayley, I know. She is often rude to me when I ask for the discharge documentation.' Her manager said okay leave it with me.

And so there was a happy ending? Well not quite. At one level nothing happened. Hayley continued with her bad behaviour and patients hung around waiting for discharge.

But something did change. Sarah's outlook and mood improved immeasurably. Importantly, the two colleagues she had asked for input treated her with a new respect and she found a much stronger bond with them.

The biggest change though was in her own head. She described the experience as: "putting the problem out there, not in here." Hayley still made the Princess jibes and Sarah found herself saying: "Oh give it a rest, the joke has worn off." Sarah used the phrase 'found myself' when she told me about this. "It just seemed to jump out of my mouth, I wasn't planning it, but I was so pleased when I said it," she said.

Over the next few months, Sarah considered her future. She was no longer obsessing over silly, sad Hayley; she had faded into the background. Sarah described her as like a noisy budgie in the corner of the room.

With that in its place she could see the issue she really needed to tackle. Her real worry was a manager who did nothing to implement a good plan and took no action to rein in a rude and obstructive employee. So she decided to look for a workplace with a more go-ahead culture and eventually ended up working for a student health service where she headed up a project on student sexual health. She says she has never been happier in her career.

***

Stories from a nursing life: Tara Beaumont

"It's about caring and you can't teach that"

Tara Beaumont spent most of her career in oncology and palliative care. She describes the rich experience of end of life care and the stresses of dealing with health organisations' politics and cultures.

When did you decide to become a nurse?
It was an organic process really, I had always wanted to be a teacher, and wanted to teach children with special needs. I chose not to go to university at 18 and so took a role as a support worker for adults with learning disabilities. I found the caring side of the role very rewarding and from there decided to do my general training. My godmother was a nurse and my grandfather's death from lung cancer influenced my choice too.

What was the appeal?
Three key aspects appealed to me, I could care for people in need, this has always been an important part of who I am. Nursing offered me a way to combine this, with an academic structure and career pathway.

How did you take the decision - alone, with help from friends, family or a careers adviser?
Family and friends were key to supporting my decision,

although there were some raised eyebrows as I can be a bit squeamish at times!

Did you consider any other careers? If so, what were they and why did you reject them?
Careers advice at school wanted me to consider being a secretary, but being in an office all day wasn't for me, and even though I have had roles which have meant I have spent significant time at a desk, I still prefer to be out and about. Teaching really appealed, and it's something I have enjoyed as a nurse.

How did you decide which branch of nursing to go into?
The death of my grandfather from lung cancer influenced me greatly, and while training I supported myself by working as a support worker looking after people approaching the end of their life in their own homes, many of whom had cancer.

Did you have an image or fantasy about what nursing would be like?
I didn't have any romantic images of nursing, that it was all lovely and about being kind to everyone. The stories my godmother told me never left me in any doubt that it is hard work, physically and emotionally.

What were the highs and lows of being a nursing student when you trained?
Well certainly a low point was finding on my first ward placement that nursing auxiliaries were terrifying to work with!!

Two in particular ran the ward, with disregard for the qualified nurses, sadly I learnt very little positive on that first placement. Luckily for me most other placements were better, although only a couple could be described as very good. Often I felt an extra pair of hands and learning was secondary.

The highlight for me was twofold, I was able to travel to America for a six-week internship, my focus was oncology and that experience has stayed with me throughout my career. Second was my placement to the local cancer centre, where my supported learning was excellent.

How did your career develop post qualification?
My career progressed from staff nurse, to sister and then to clinical nurse specialist.

My focus was oncology and palliative care. I spent a few years in acute oncology to gain experience in the area. However, my passion has always been palliative care. I worked in hospitals and the community and spent 10 years with the UK charity Breast Cancer Care, which enabled me to use my nursing skills in very varied way, utilising social media, patient information, health care professional teaching and influencing policy nationally and locally.

My last post was with the Macmillan community palliative care team in Barnsley as a CNS, it was a role I truly loved and was very sad to leave due to my ill health.

Who have been the most important role models during your career? What qualities did you most admire in them?
My first preceptor; for her compassion towards both her patients and her colleagues and the fact that she had time for everyone. I took that through all my career, it is very important that nurses have time.

What has been the biggest challenge for you as a nurse?
The politics in both the NHS and in other healthcare settings. You can spend so much time protecting your own

department then there are so many egos to deal with. Often the balance seems wrong and patient care isn't the centre as it should be.

Did you ever feel that the demands of the job put you under unacceptably high levels of stress?
Yes, very much so.

How did you deal with that?
In early days very badly. Even as I progressed I felt I could have dealt with it better.

I think it is wrong that there is no specific training or preparation in coping with the sort of pressure which nursing brings, also there is still a culture that it is what you should expect, which makes it difficult to say that you are struggling.

Working in oncology and palliative care, there is often an assumption that it is the nature of the job which is causing the pressure. I must say I never felt that, it was much more about the politics and the culture. I loved the patient contact and often felt I could take refuge in looking after the patients.

What strategies did you use to get you through the most challenging times in your career?
Role models are so important. I think having some role models and trusted people who you can really talk to and who share the same values as you makes all the difference.

What are you most proud of in terms of your career as a nurse?
I once received a letter from a patient's family after she had died. Her husband said he feared that as I got more senior I would move away from direct patient care and that

would be such a shame. It really influenced me and I made sure I never did that. I never moved away from patients.

What would you say is the most important quality needed to be a good nurse?
To care. And you can't teach it.

In your opinion, how has nursing changed since you were starting out?
It has become more academic, this is a good thing. However the general public's perception of nursing has changed and often not for the better. We have more professional status than when I started, but compared with the United States we are still not considered in the same professional light.

Would you recommend nursing to anyone considering a career in the profession today?
I'm not sure. Because it is a very hard life. You have to be a certain sort of person and have that ability to care. If you have that then it can be very good indeed.

Key Facts

When did you train as a nurse?
March 1992-March 1995, but I worked as a support worker from 1989

Where?
I trained in Sheffield

Qualifications
Registered Nurse (Adult), Diploma in nursing studies which I then converted to a BSc. (Hons) degree with the Open University and I have an MSc. in supportive and palliative care. I also have ENB 237 (oncology), 998 (teaching course) (HIV and Aids) E111 (Breast Care Nurse) and a certificate in counselling.

Current role
I am retired from nursing and currently own and manage a gardening business with my husband who is a retired police officer

Chapter Eight
Looking after yourself: eating well when it's hard

There is an irony that places where we should be pushing the healthy eating message are often toxic food environments. Here are some ideas about how you can change this and some examples of good practice.

As a nurse you are well-informed about nutrition and exercise, so I am not going to waste your time telling you what you already know.

Instead I am going to concentrate on why it is so difficult as a nurse to maintain a healthy eating pattern, and what you can do to change that.

So, what is the problem?
We have already looked at the damage shift work can do, but on top of that there is the lack of healthy foods on hospital sites, missed meal breaks, long working hours which can mean you are too tired to make a proper meal when you get home, and often a hospital culture of grateful patients and their families using foods (especially chocolates) as a thank you.

In 2009 the Department of Health estimated that 700,000 of its staff were either overweight or obese. Yet only 19 per cent of NHS trusts in London had a healthy eating policy and only eight percent had a physical activity policy for staff. The UK government of 2010-2015 issued guidance that hospital canteens must offer food which complies with the government's own recommendations on the amount of sugar and fat in food[1], but too many hospitals still have the coffee chains and the vending machines full of crisps.

There have been some local initiatives which have shown the way. Cambridgeshire's Hinchingbrooke Hospital's restaurant even won a gold catering mark from the Soil Association for the quality of its food (to date, the only hospital in the UK to have achieved this). But even this bright spark only had day-time opening hours and these are shortened even further at the weekends.[2]

The Soil Association has a good track record of supporting healthy eating in hospitals. It issued a report in 2011 which detailed some best practice and found that where hospitals sourced food locally they often saved money.[3]

In 2016 the chief executive of NHS England, Simon Stevens, pledged to introduce a sugar tax in hundreds of acute, mental health and community services hospitals by 2020 and in every local health centre. He also promised to use the proceeds to improve the health of NHS workers.

These are welcome changes, but the day to day reality can still be tough so I am going to suggest a few ways that you can get the best out of what is often an unhealthy situation.

Get in the eating habit
Routine counts; if you miss meals your blood sugar will be all over the place. Bad eating patterns can trigger increasing triglyceride production which is then stored as body fat and can add to your weight. So what do you do when you cannot

get a meal break? This is the time when you will be tempted to eat unhealthy high calorie snacks.

Try to keep this emergency supply pack for when you have to miss a meal.

Emergency pack: Your 5-minute meal
Water (keep hydrated)
Seeds
Nuts
High protein shake (if you have access to a fridge)
Vegetable batons or a piece of fruit
Small piece of cheese

Eat little and often
If you have a 12-hour shift ahead of you and suspect you may not get a proper break it is tempting to eat a big meal before you start. This is not the best way, you may overload your system and end up beginning the shift feeling bloated and tired. It is better to have a variety of small snacks which you can pace throughout the shift.

Set yourself some rules
The fast food outlets and vending machines all over our hospitals are there to make profits for the private companies that run them; they are not primarily interested in your health and wellbeing or that of your patients. Avoid them, make your own choices and you will be healthier and save money.

Water, water – make it a rule to only drink water in the working day – avoid caffeine, (remember it is in fizzy drinks as well as coffee) as it may mean you have difficult sleeping later in the day.

No going to the vending machine and grabbing crisps and a chocolate bar. Make it a rule never to do it and make sure you have the materials for the 5-minute meal above.

When you do your weekly shop buy fruit, nuts and vegetables. Keep these at work to grab in those really rushed times. You can add high-protein bars, but check the labels as some are full of sugar.

Breathe

Breathe before eating. If you are stressed you will not digest food properly. So take a few moments (all you need is a few moments) and do some diaphragmatic breathing, counting breaths before you eat anything. Get you colleagues involved – all breathe together and no giggling!

Check if you are hungry

It is easy to use food as a pick me up if you are tired at work or just to mark the fact you have a short break. Stop for a moment and check if you are actually hungry – you may just be thirsty. Make sure you take a drink of water and then see if you still feel hungry. If you are not hungry mark the break or deal with the tiredness in another way. Go outside for some fresh air. Do your breathing exercises again. Or do this 3-minute refresher – it will energise and calm you. Take a few seconds when you have finished this to feel how much better you feel. It works doesn't it?

3-minute refresher

Go somewhere quiet, sit if you can but if you have to stand that is okay.
1. Imagine a glass ball on the top of your head, you have to balance it so keep very still.
2. This ball is filled with a magic refreshing substance. It is coloured. Imagine its colour.
3. Imagine the glass ball opens and the magic substance enters the top of your head. It is cool (or warm – you choose)

4. It slowly moves down your body like a wave. It enters every fibre of your body.
5. Feel it moving down right to your toes.
6. When it gets there, stretch
7. Breathe deeply

Change the food culture on your ward

We live in a culture where we use sweet unhealthy food as a reward in various ways and this culture is very strong in healthcare settings. It won't change overnight, but if it feels right in your workplace you might consider doing something about it. There are rewards which are not a box of chocolates!

Here are a few suggestions which have come from work I have done with nurses who wanted to lose weight. This meant we had to come up with some ways they could cope with the biscuits and sweets culture on the ward. Not all these ideas will fit your circumstances but some might and you may think of other changes which suit your workplace culture.

The new fruit challenge

I know of a few instances where nurses have stood up and said 'no more biscuits on the ward' and insisted on fresh fruit instead. To make it fun, you can try to get unusual fruit as well as the usual apples, you can even set up a challenge – everyone on the ward has to eat a fruit they have never tasted before each month. This will get you all thinking about what unusual fruits you have never tasted and where you can get them.

Charity donations

If patients are giving you sweets to show their appreciation perhaps you could encourage a charity donation instead? Can you make some posters or leaflets to give the patients and their relatives – "We're getting healthy so PLEASE don't give us sweets – if you want to say thanks then we are partnering with (your chosen charity)." You can then give a nice thank you card or note to any patients who contribute to your chosen charity.

Birthday treats

Do you have a culture where people bring in cakes on their birthday? There are healthier and more enjoyable ways to celebrate. If you have a music system in your staff room then why not start a tradition of everyone bringing in their favourite music on their birthday? Or, if that doesn't fit your circumstances, what about counting up all that money spent on cakes over the year and putting the money towards an 'it's our ward birthday' or 'it's all our birthdays' spa day or trip to a favourite place once a year (or more often!).

References

(1)
https://www.gov.uk/government/news/new-rules-to-serve-up-better-food-for-nhs-patients-and-staff)
(2)
http://www.hinchingbrooke.nhs.uk/patients-and-visitors/restaurants-and-shop/
(3)
http://www.soilassociation.org/LinkClick.aspx?fileticket=2p%2Fa nl11%2B6o%3D&tabid=388

Chapter Nine

Looking after yourself: building good networks

Can you develop a mindset that will enable you to get the very best from your colleagues? In most cases the answer is 'yes if you know how'. And it will make you happier and more effective.

Working at the frontline of human experience can be draining as well as exhilarating. And on top of that your work can be literally life and death. That's some responsibility to carry day in day out, so you need good support if you are going to feel happy and confident and able to cope with whatever comes up day on day.

I want to talk in this chapter about the sort of professional frameworks and support which can provide you with a safety net when you need it and also help you develop your knowledge, come up with new solutions to problems and generally help you feel good about yourself and your professional competence.

So let's start by looking at supervision
I regard good supervision as the gold standard of professional support. I am myself a trained and accredited supervisor, so I see its benefits everyday as I supervise

practitioners who offer a variety of talking therapies. I also know from my clients who work in healthcare settings that those who have good supervision in place usually cope better and develop faster. Supervision can be invaluable where difficulties and risks arise and so is a great safety net. It is evident that where we have seen scandals about care, good supervision has usually been missing.

But it is not just in crisis or danger situations that supervision has value. A time set aside, in a positive and non-judgemental environment, where you can examine even routine tasks and actions and discuss how you could do them better can help you be a happier person and a better nurse.

Supervision is an unfortunate name, with its connotations of management oversight and direction. Actually good supervision should be the exact opposite of this.

My work as a supervisor for other therapists is one of the most rewarding things I do. It's the best place in the world to help another professional grow and learn and begin to reach conclusions for themselves about their practice.

After a session, they nearly always have a clearer idea about what they can do better and, just as important, what they already do well, and they leave the session with a spring in their step. It is a creative process on both sides. Where it works, it helps you learn from your knowledge and feelings and practice and then offer an even better service. What's not to like about that?

So supervision is structured discussion where you get the chance to review and reflect on your work and how you could do it even better. It's not about dwelling on mistakes or apportioning blame. It starts with the assumption that you are a responsible professional with the skills and knowledge to deliver excellent care. It's about fostering a mental attitude which is constantly looking for new solutions to current issues.[1]

Organisations that concern themselves with improving patient care and protecting standards are generally very supportive of clinical supervision. For example, The Care Quality Commission says clinical supervision should provide staff with the opportunity to:
• Reflect on and review their practice
• Discuss individual cases in depth
• Change or modify their practice and identify training and continuing development needs.

The Commission's guidance suggests: "It can help staff to manage the personal and professional demands created by the nature of their work.

"This is particularly important for those who work with people who have complex and challenging needs – clinical supervision provides an environment in which they can explore their own personal and emotional reactions to their work. It can allow the member of staff to reflect on and challenge their own practice in a safe and confidential environment. They can also receive feedback that is separate from managerial considerations."[2]

The Nursing and Midwifery Council also supports supervision. It identifies the possible benefits of receiving effective clinical supervision as: "Improved capacity to identify solutions to problems, increased understanding of professional issues, improved standards of patient care, opportunities to further develop skills and knowledge and enhanced understanding of own practice."[3]

So how do you get good supervision?
There is no one model or protocol for supervision in the NHS and private employers may not offer supervision at all. Provision is a bit of a patchwork. The rules also differ from country to country so we have quite a complicated mish-mash to find our way through.

If you are a practising nurse, you can expect to receive clinical supervision. It should not be used as a management tool to deliver external targets and it should not be a box-ticking exercise. The intention is to help you reflect on how you do your work and learn both from your mistakes and from what you did well. Because arrangements and types of supervision differ between individual trusts and workplaces, the advice I am giving has to be quite general.

Models of supervision
My aim is to give you some pointers about getting the most out of your supervision and to provide some information which will help you to improve things if you feel that what you are getting falls short. Even if you are not always in full control of your supervision, I hope you can still make some choices which help you. There are different forms of supervision and ways to do supervision, but most successful models are solution-focused. That means they take an issue or a difficulty and look at how it would be if that problem was solved and what it would take to make that happen. This almost always involves looking at different aspects of complex situations.

Many of the best models for supervision derive from nursing. One of my favourites is from Barbara Carper, who identifies four 'patterns of knowing'.

This four-pattern model is very useful for enabling you to work with the truth that your work is more than just facts and science. This is especially important as modern nursing is increasingly based on measuring outcomes and evidence-base and it is important that human emotion is not left out.

Carper acknowledges the importance of factual knowledge, based on empirically verified science as one 'pattern of knowing'. Then she goes on to talk about the other forms of knowledge. These are the personal, derived from self-understanding and being empathetic with patients; ethical, an awareness of moral questions and choices; and aesthetic (in the sense of 'relating to the here and now') which takes account of all aspects of the patient's experience.

So what makes supervision work?

First of all, get a good supervisor. I hope you have some choice over this; it is good practice to allow a supervisee to choose a supervisor and it is important that you have a supervisor with whom you can build a good rapport and who you respect and trust.

Your supervisor should have received specific training in supervision. It is not an easy thing to deliver; to supervise others well your supervisor needs a complex set of skills including building rapport, developing reflective practice, solution-focused questioning and risk management.

Ideally, your supervisor should also be outside of your mainstream management structure, remember supervision is not formal performance review or an evaluation process. It is important that you feel you can be completely open and honest with your supervisor. Everything you say should be completely confidential (with the proviso that your supervisor can take action if they feel you or those in your care are at serious risk).

If possible, it is good practice to draw up a contract before beginning supervision. Discuss how often sessions will take place and how long they will last. Get in place some 'emergency' arrangements in case there comes a time when you feel you are faced with a situation which is damaging your well-being and your ability to work well with your patients.

So what does a good supervision session look like? As you are dealing with complex situations there will be a huge range of subjects which can be covered, but you should emerge with a clearer insight into what you did, why you did it and what you can do in the future.

Here are some questions and points which you may use to evaluate your supervision sessions. After the session do you have:

• A knowledge and understanding of how you work when you are *not* encountering problems, and an idea of how you could replicate this in areas where you do find difficulties.

• An insight into what your client or patient is feeling in a particular situation.

• Insight into what (in difficult situations) you could do instead?

• Some guidance and understanding of how you can learn any new skills you need; how you can monitor your own performance and how you can evaluate how you are doing, and how you feel.

How does a solution-focused supervision session work?
I've talked quite a bit about solution-focus, so I'll try to explain that a bit more by describing how I conduct my own supervision sessions.

At the start of the session I always ask the supervisee how they are. This often involves asking what has gone well and if there is any client contact which they feel has gone badly.

I then ask the supervisee what is their goal in coming to supervision today and what they would like to achieve. I also ask them what would have to happen for them to consider the session worthwhile. This gives a structure to the session which reflects their wishes. I then question the supervisee, asking what they feel went well in the situation we are discussing, and what they might do differently. As the conversation develops it may be that my supervisee recognises a skills or knowledge gap and we can talk about how that can be addressed. Or the supervisee might recognise that, in fact, they performed much better than they thought they had (this is very common, most of us lack confidence and are very ready to be self-critical).

I might then ask when the supervisee feels confident and when not – perhaps we discover that he or she has a relationship with a particular manager which is less than satisfactory and we can discuss how that can be improved. Or we might identify a skills gap or a preference for a certain sort of working environment. All of this is adding to the self-knowledge which can both improve practice and make you happier.

The supervisee's wellbeing is important so I will be keeping an eye out for signs of burnout and stress. Supervision sessions can have a training element. I sometimes offer advice and techniques which can be used to help protect mental wellbeing when faced with a difficult situation.

I encourage my supervisees to keep a reflective diary. This means they can record for themselves what happened in the session and any goals they have set. It can also be helpful to scale how useful they found the session and how they feel about themselves and their practice.

Group supervision
Often you will be offered group supervision and this can be a great way of developing really strong teams.

If you are asked to participate in group supervision, ask how the ground rules for sessions will be set and if you have any choice in the membership of the group.

Group supervision can be fantastically powerful as it gives the chance to look at situations from different perspectives, but it only works if all the participants trust each other and have broad agreement on what the supervision sessions are for. It goes without saying that confidentiality must be maintained.

Building your professional networks
Apart from formal supervision, there are other professional structures which can help you have a happy and fulfilled working life. Strong professional networks can be anything from a structured peer group which meets regularly, to just meeting up in the pub for a drink after work once a week.

Face to face peer support
There is some evidence that peer support groups help nurses resist burnout and stress. A study in the *Journal of Advanced Nursing* found that problem-based peer support had a significant role in alleviating stress. Those participating in the study felt the group gave them increased self confidence, knowledge and a sense of belonging.

Confidence may be the key factor here. Confidence gives you the ability to take control of your work and your potential. Support helps you gain that confidence. In other words, you need your professional mates around you.

The key thing is a space to talk to others who understand what you do and with whom you can share experiences and debate issues in a non-judgemental and supportive way. Make building your networks a professional task from day one. If you are a student make sure you keep in contact with the people you like when you finish, and similarly when you move jobs in the future.

Using social media
Face-to-face contact is special and if you can make time to develop a face-to-face network, even if it is informal, then you will almost certainly benefit. But this is not always possible, and social media can be a wonderful alternative.

Online groups work best where people have an offline relationship as well, or where they have developed after an initial face-to-face.

So, you could set up a small closed group on Facebook with, for example people you trained with or people you met at a conference or in a union meeting. If you want the group to grow, you could allow others to then invite professionals who they know, either directly through work or through other professional networks. This way you can build a sizeable and diverse online network, but still have the security of knowing that your online contacts have all been recommended by a real person working in a real workplace or in a real social network.

This should keep out trolls and troublemakers. Do remember though to keep your personal and your professional interactions on Facebook separate.

If you don't want to set up a group yourself, you may find existing groups that suit your needs on LinkedIn. Getting started is simple, just join LinkedIn and then search for nurses' groups. They will have an administrator and it is worth messaging the administrator of the group to introduce yourself and ask if they discuss the sort of things which interest you.

Both LinkedIn and Facebook are free. The only thing they will take is your time.

Multi-professional networks
Whether offline or online, it is worth extending your professional network beyond just nursing, based on what you do and where you want your career to go. For example, if you work as a school nurse you may want to reach out to people in the education world or who run local youth services. If you are a cancer nurse, you may find contact with a local cancer charity is useful professionally.

193

If you plan to work in another country at some stage it is worth looking for online groups of nurses based in that country. This can prepare you well for the differences you may find should you take the plunge and decide to nurse abroad.

References
1
Reflecting peer-support groups in the prevention of stress and burnout: randomized controlled trial
Ulla Peterson1, *et al*
Article first published online: 11 Aug 2008
Accessed Feb 2016
http://www.ncbi.nlm.nih.gov/pubmed/18727753
2
Care Quality Commission (2013) Supporting Information and Guidance: Supporting Effective Clinical Supervision. London: Care Quality Commission
3 Nursing and Midwifery Council (2008) The Code – Standards of Conduct, Performance and Ethics to Nurses and Midwives. London: Nursing and Midwifery Council

Index

Index

Index

Index

Afterword from Ann

If you want to put the ideas from this book into practice I will help you set up a readers' club.

Christine Hancock expressed a very interesting thought in her foreword for this book. She said: "My concern is whether busy nurses will find this book? Will they have time to read it? Will they be able to act upon the ideas, advice and suggestions that could be important to them? She went on to suggest: "Perhaps groups of nurses might share it? Each concentrating on one or two aspects and use it to stimulate discussion."

I pondered on this and discussed it with some of my colleagues and came up with the idea of a nurses' bookclub or reading group where you can use this book to support each other.

So this is my idea of how this could work

As soon as you set up a reading group, contact me via the website and I will do these things for you

• I will give you a discount code so your group members will get the book at a lower price.

- I will send you special extra materials not available to anyone else.
- You can email me and ask me a question which has arisen from your reader sessions.
- I will also host a group Skype session for your group on any subject covered in the book.

Ideas for readers' club sessions
You can use the book exactly as you want, but if you are not sure here are some suggestions of the sort of sessions you could hold.
- Your work and your lives – what makes you happiest and how can you increase that?
- Burnout, have you suffered – what did you do?
- Career changes – where do you want to go, how will things change for you? What's it like working in a different setting?
- Shift work – share your secrets for coping.
- Looking after yourself eating and exercising, supporting each other.

And finally, I'm asking a favour from you. Now you have read the book, can you let me know what I left out? If you tell me I will try my best to write it and keep you updated.

Visit our website

As a valued reader you can access a lot more resources.

We are constantly posting new information on topics

such as anxiety management, smoking cessation,

nutrition and exercise. And we have self help tools and

audio downloads as well. Go to

www.nursesbook.com

And enter the password nh 6458

the nurses' handbook

www.ingramcontent.com/pod-product-compliance
Lightning Source LLC
Chambersburg PA
CBHW060020210326
41520CB00009B/947